Introduction to Musculoskeletal Ultrasound

Introduction to Musculoskeletal Ultrasound

Getting Started

JEFFREY A. STRAKOWSKI, MD

Clinical Associate Professor
Department of Physical Medicine and Rehabilitation
Ohio State University School of Medicine
Columbus, Ohio

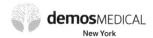

demosMEDICAL

New York

Visit our website at www.demosmedical.com

ISBN: 9781620700655
e-book ISBN: 9781617052309

Acquisitions Editor: Beth Barry
Compositor: diacriTech, Chennai

Medicine is an ever-changing science. Research and clinical experience are continually expanding our knowledge, in particular our understanding of proper treatment and drug therapy. The authors, editors, and publisher have made every effort to ensure that all information in this book is in accordance with the state of knowledge at the time of production of the book. Nevertheless, the authors, editors, and publisher are not responsible for errors or omissions or for any consequences from application of the information in this book and make no warranty, expressed or implied, with respect to the contents of the publication. Every reader should examine carefully the package inserts accompanying each drug and should carefully check whether the dosage schedules mentioned therein or the contraindications stated by the manufacturer differ from the statements made in this book. Such examination is particularly important with drugs that are either rarely used or have been newly released on the market.

Library of Congress Cataloging-in-Publication Data
Strakowski, Jeffrey A., author.
 Introduction to musculoskeletal ultrasound: getting started / Jeffrey A. Strakowski.
    p. ; cm.
 Includes bibliographical references and index.
 ISBN 978-1-62070-065-5—ISBN 978-1-61705-230-9 (e-Book)
 I. Title.
 [DNLM: 1. Musculoskeletal System—ultrasonography. 2. Ultrasonography—methods. WE 141]
 RC925.7
 616.7'07543—dc23
                    2015028595

Special discounts on bulk quantities of Demos Medical Publishing books are available to corporations, professional associations, pharmaceutical companies, health care organizations, and other qualifying groups. For details, please contact:

Special Sales Department
Demos Medical Publishing, LLC
11 West 42nd Street, 15th Floor
New York, NY 10036
Phone: 800-532-8663 or 212-683-0072
Fax: 212-941-7842
E-mail: specialsales@demosmedical.com

Printed in the United States of America by Bradford & Bigelow.
15 16 17 18 / 5 4 3 2 1

To my family—Danielle, Nathan, Devin, and Hannah for their love, support, and tolerance.

Also to my residents whose excitement for learning helped inspire the creation of the book.

Contents

Preface   ix
Acknowledgments   xi

  1. Introduction   1

  2. Physics of Ultrasound   3

  3. Understanding the Equipment   17

  4. Image Optimization   41

  5. Scanning Techniques and Ergonomics   51

  6. Doppler Imaging   61

  7. Imaging Tendon   69

  8. Imaging Muscle   81

  9. Imaging Nerve   99

10. Imaging of Other Tissues   115

11. Imaging Masses   141

12. Foreign Bodies   149

13. Artifacts   155

14. Ultrasound Guidance for Injections   165

15. Developing a Clinical Practice   179

Index   *183*

Preface

The use of high frequency ultrasound as an imaging modality for the musculoskeletal system has expanded dramatically in the past decade. Technological advancements have led to progressively improving image resolution and a broader scope of applications. The value of ultrasound in improving diagnostic acumen and safety and accuracy in dynamic guidance of interventional procedures has resulted in increased use in musculoskeletal clinics.

Despite its growth, standardized training for use of this modality is not yet available in the majority of residency training programs. The number of qualified instructors has increased over the years, leading to the speculation that formal instruction in musculoskeletal ultrasound will develop in both residencies and medical schools. The increasing recognition of its value has also resulted in more education in musculoskeletal ultrasound for sonographers.

This text was written in an effort to illustrate and teach the basic components of many of the skills and knowledge needed to begin incorporating the use of ultrasound in a musculoskeletal practice. A concern often expressed by both my resident physicians and established practitioners who attended our didactic courses was that attempting to get started was very intimidating. They often cited that learning the skills needed to operate the equipment and obtain and interpret the images appears too daunting and that many of the available courses and texts initially appear too advanced.

The goal of this book is to provide a simplified approach for those getting started in musculoskeletal ultrasound. This includes developing understanding in use of the controls and function of the ultrasound machine, commonly used terminology, obtaining and optimizing the image, and proper scanning technique. It also is designed to instruct in the recognition of the appearance of various musculoskeletal tissue, commonly seen artifacts, foreign bodies and masses, and understanding basics of interventional ultrasound. Principles of further advancement of skills and initiating a practice are also discussed. The chapters contain concise instructional concepts, a large number of illustrations to assist with understanding, and helpful reminders summarizing the key educational points.

It has been exciting to watch the growth of interest in this field. It is my hope that this text can help beginners make the first steps into the rapidly growing knowledge base of musculoskeletal ultrasound and ultimately develop more advanced learning and progression of skills.

Jeffrey A. Strakowski, MD

Acknowledgments

I would like to thank the physicians and staff at Physical Medicine Associates and the McConnell Spine, Sport and Joint Center, and the residents and faculty in the department of Physical Medicine and Rehabilitation at The Ohio State University for their support in this work.

I would also like to acknowledge General Electric, Sonosite, and CAE Health Care whose products were used in the creation of many of the images.

Introduction

The decision to get started in the discipline of musculoskeletal ultrasound is not an easy one. Individuals embarking on this endeavor often have no prior experience in the use of ultrasound and understanding the images and instrumentation can be daunting. This is coupled with the fact that there is often no standardized training available and considerable academic rigor is needed to develop proficiency in the use of ultrasound of the musculoskeletal system.

Ultrasound has become an increasingly popular tool for visualizing soft tissue in all areas of medicine. It provides a number of advantages over other imaging modalities. It provides real-time imaging that does not rely on ionizing radiation and can be used in the presence of metallic implants. There are no issues with claustrophobia and no reliance on immobile-imaging centers. There are no known adverse effects with the use of diagnostic ultrasound and therefore, no specific restrictions. Additional advantages of ultrasound include dynamic visualization with the ability to see moving tissue. This can be invaluable in circumstances where dynamic abnormalities might go unrecognized in static images. Doppler imaging is also available on most ultrasound machines, which allows real-time assessment of vascular flow. This is valuable when assessing both normal and pathologic vascularity.

Ultrasound is an ideal modality for needle guidance for many diagnostic and therapeutic procedures. It allows real-time visualization of needle motion in conjunction with the target and surrounding soft tissue structures. Acquiring needle guidance skills with ultrasound can greatly enhance safety and accuracy with needle procedures.

The development of high-resolution broadband high-frequency transducers has led to vast improvements in visualization of the relatively superficial structures in the musculoskeletal system. As a result, ultrasound can provide information not always available with other imaging modalities. The acumen provided by this information can be beneficial to any musculoskeletal practice. The relatively low cost, portability, and instant feedback of results also greatly enhances patient satisfaction.

Once the decision is made to develop skills in high-frequency ultrasound, a plan is needed for obtaining appropriate equipment and learning how to use it. Currently, there are limited formal training programs for musculoskeletal ultrasound in residency. Online instruction is available; however, there is no replacement for hands-on instruction. This can be found in many courses offered around the country and world. The current trends suggest that there will be an increase in learning opportunities in medical schools and residency programs.

As with any skill, many hours of practice are needed to develop proficiency. An examiner needs familiarity with the instrumentation and image optimization as well as proper scanning techniques and ergonomics. Recognition of characteristic tissue appearance and their changes in pathologic conditions is required to perform a competent musculoskeletal ultrasound examination. Knowledge of artifacts and minimizing their impact on the image is also necessary.

Incorporation of ultrasound into clinical practice is also challenging. It is particularly daunting for individuals already beyond their formal training and in established practice. Greater resources are becoming available to assist with education and skill development, clinical competency, and coding and billing. It takes the development of a substantial knowledge base and countless hours of practice to perform effective musculoskeletal ultrasound, but the results can be greatly rewarding.

2

Physics of Ultrasound

A comprehensive review of the physics used in ultrasonography is beyond the scope of this text. Despite this, some understanding of the basic physics used in ultrasound is needed for optimal creation and interpretation of an ultrasound image. Ultrasound images are created by reflected sound waves returning back to the transducer. The nature of the image is based on the properties of different tissues in the body. There are a number of factors that influence this process.

PIEZOELECTRIC EFFECT

Piezoelectricity was first discovered by Pierre and Jacques Curie in 1880 using natural quartz. Ultrasound machines use the piezoelectric effect to generate an image. The *piezoelectric effect* refers to the creation of electrical energy by applying another energy (pressure) to a crystal. The word *piezo* is derived from the Greek word that means pressure. In the case of ultrasound, this is defined by the generation of sound waves emitted from the transducer crystals when precise electrical charges are applied to make them vibrate. The sound waves given off by the transducer is also known as the *pulse*. This process is known as the *reverse (or inverse) piezoelectric effect*. The direct piezoelectric effect occurs when the electrical potentials are created by the effect on the crystals from the sound waves returning to the transducer from the tissue. This is also known as the *echo*. The distinct pattern of electrical charges, given off by returning sound waves, is used to create the image on the ultrasound screen.

SOUND WAVES

Frequency

Frequency of the sound wave is measured in cycles per second or Hertz (Hz).

By definition, sound waves greater than 20,000 Hz are in the ultrasonic range. They are considered ultrasonic because they are outside of the normal human range of hearing, which is 20 to 20,000 Hz. The frequency used in medical ultrasound imaging is generally 2 to 15 megahertz (MHz). The range for most superficial musculoskeletal applications is at the higher end of this, generally 8 to 15 MHz.

The frequency of the emitted sound wave is controlled by the design of the transducer (Figure 2.1). Most transducers are described by the range they are capable of emitting. This range is termed the *bandwidth* of the transducer. Transducers that have more than one range of operating frequencies are called *broad bandwidth transducers*.

Image optimization requires attention to frequency. Lower frequency sound waves penetrate more deeply and therefore, can provide better clarity of a deeper structure (Figure 2.2). By contrast, higher frequency sound waves do not penetrate tissue as well but provide higher resolution of a more superficial structure (Figure 2.3).

Attenuation

As sound waves travel through tissue, there is a progressive reduction in the intensity of the wave. This process is known as *attenuation* (Figure 2.4). Note that over a given distance, higher frequency sound waves generally

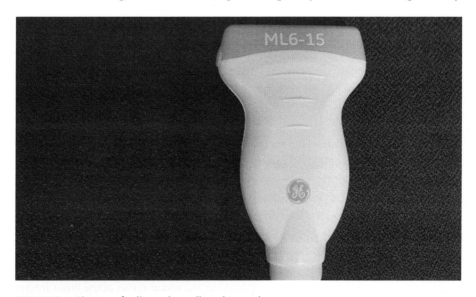

FIGURE 2.1 Picture of a linear broadband transducer.

High frequency
waveform

Low frequency
waveform

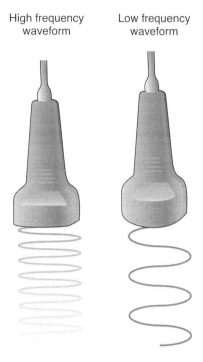

FIGURE 2.2 Illustration demonstrating the difference between high-frequency and low-frequency ultrasonic waveforms. Note that the low-frequency waveform penetrates deeper in the same tissue. High-frequency waveforms provide better resolution of more superficial tissue.

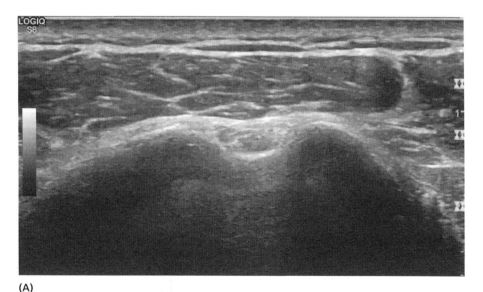

(A)

FIGURE 2.3 Sonograms demonstrating the effect of incident sound wave frequency changes on the appearance of the image. The frequencies shown are at (A) 15 MHz, (B) 12 MHz, (C) 9 MHz, and (D) 8 MHz. Although the differences might appear relatively minimal, there is a better resolution of the superficial structures at the higher frequencies and better penetration of the sound waves at the lower frequencies.

(continued)

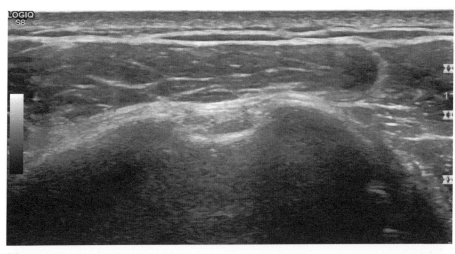

(B)

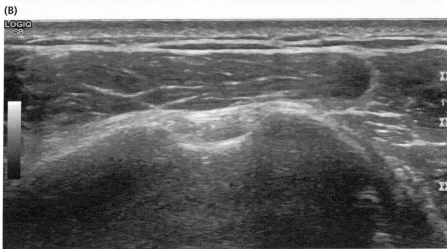

(C)

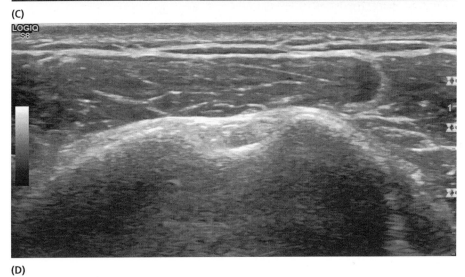

(D)

FIGURE 2.3 *(continued)*

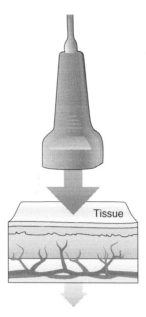

FIGURE 2.4 Illustration demonstrating attenuation of the incident sound waves (red arrow) as it travels through tissue. The continuing propagating sound wave is smaller due to the reflection, refraction, and absorption of portions of the incident sound wave.

have more attenuation than lower frequency waves. The attenuation occurs as a result of three processes: *reflection, refraction,* and *absorption.* The property of the degree of sound wave attenuation in specific tissue is known as that tissue's *attenuation coefficient.*

Reflection

Reflection in ultrasound refers to the return of the sound wave energy back to the transducer. This principle is what allows the image to be generated by the ultrasound machine. Generally, more reflection results in a more hyperechoic (brighter) image. Reflection occurs at tissue boundaries where the tissues on either side of the boundaries have differences in *acoustic impedance* (Figure 2.5). Larger differences in these acoustic impendences, therefore, result in more reflection. The reflection can be considered either specular or diffuse. Specular reflection occurs when the sound waves encounter large smooth surfaces such as bone, which results in the sound waves being reflected back in a relatively uniform direction. The cells of most soft tissue create a more diffuse pattern of reflection to the transducer (Figure 2.6).

The *angle of incidence* of the entering sound wave is also critical to the amount of reflection back to the transducer (Figure 2.7). The angle of incidence refers to the angle of deviation from a perpendicular line to the surface of the tissue. Therefore, the desired orthogonal incident wave in

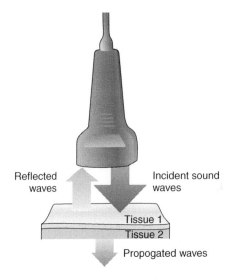

FIGURE 2.5 Illustration demonstrating reflection. A portion of the incident sound waves (red arrow) are reflected back to the transducer (green arrow) after striking tissue types with different impedance. A portion of the incident sound waves continues to propagate through the tissue (purple arrow).

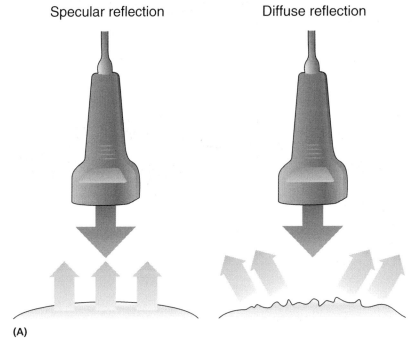

(A)

FIGURE 2.6 (A) Illustration of specular versus diffuse reflection. The smooth surface in specular reflection results in more return of the reflected sound waves to the transducer (green arrows) creating a more hyperechoic (brighter) image. The less uniform tissue in diffuse reflection results in less return of the reflected sound waves and a more hypoechoic (darker) image. (B) Sonogram showing the appearance of specular reflection. Note that the large smooth surface of the bone (yellow arrows) leads to a bright signal due to the significant impedance difference between it and the surrounding tissue. (C) Sonogram showing the appearance of more diffuse reflection in muscle tissue. Note that the smaller differences in acoustic impedance reflect various shades of gray rather than the bright signal noted with the interface of bone.

(continued)

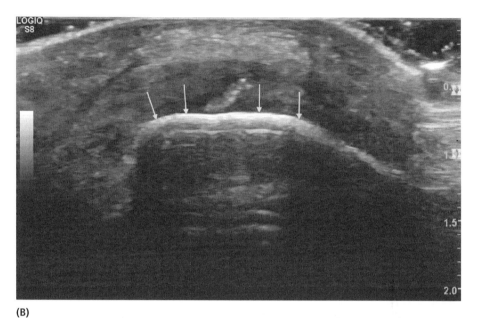

(B)

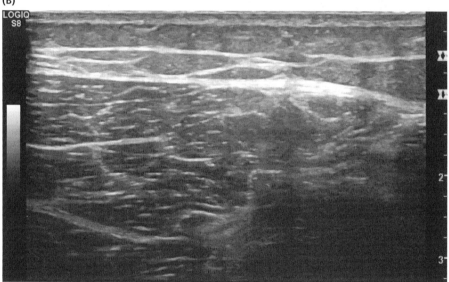

(C)

FIGURE 2.6 *(continued)*

ultrasound should be considered to have an angle of incidence of zero. When the angle of incidence is greater, fewer sound waves are reflected back to the transducer resulting in a more hypoechoic (darker) image with less clarity. The optimal reflection with the most sound waves occurs when the angle of incidence approaches zero and is virtually perpendicular (orthogonal) to the tissue of interest. An incident sound wave approach that deviates from perpendicular to the tissue (ie, angle of incidence less than 0°) results in an artifact known as *anisotropy*, which is discussed in more detail in Chapter 13 (Figure 2.8).

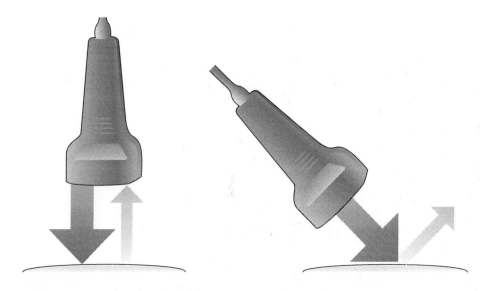

FIGURE 2.7 Illustration demonstrating the effect of the angle of incidence of the sound beam. Note that an angle of incidence that is perpendicular (ie, 0 degrees) (illustration on the left) to a smooth interface results in the largest amount of sound waves returning to the transducer. This transducer position helps create an optimum image. An incident wave hitting the interface at an angle of incidence greater than 0 degrees (ie, less than perpendicular) will result in the wave being deflected away from the transducer at an angle equal to the angle of incidence in the opposite direction (illustration on the right). In this circumstance, the signal of the returning echo is weakened creating a darker image (anisotropic artifact).

Refraction

Refraction occurs when the incident sound wave contacts the boundary of tissues at an oblique angle. This causes the reflected sound beam to travel in a direction that is away from the transducer (Figure 2.9). Refraction, therefore, results in a loss of the propagated signal. The conventional settings on the ultrasound instrumentation calculate the returning waves as though they are traveling in a straight line. This leads to a loss of image clarity as the refraction increases.

The direction of the refracted sound waves is predicted by Snell's law ($\mathrm{Sin}\,\theta_i / V_i = \mathrm{Sin}\,\theta_r / V_r$). This states that the magnitude of the refraction is directly proportional to the angle of incidence and the difference in velocity of the sound waves within the two tissue types. The relationship of the velocity characteristics of the different tissues also impacts the direction of refraction. If the propagating sound wave is faster in the first tissue because of less tissue impedance, the refraction will be more perpendicular. If the impedance is less in the second tissue with resultant faster sound wave propagation, refraction occurs away from the original direction (Figure 2.9).

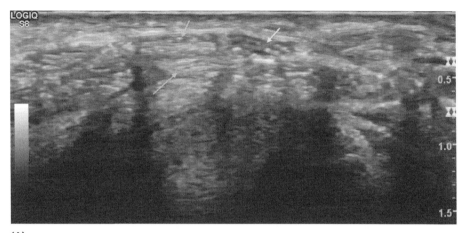

(A)

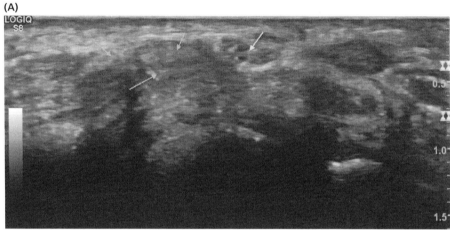

(B)

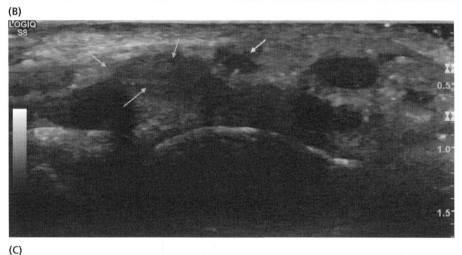

(C)

FIGURE 2.8 Sonograms demonstrating the effect of anisotropic artifact on the image. The median nerve (yellow arrow) is shown in proximity to surrounding flexor tendons (blue arrows). In (A), the incident sound beam is close to orthogonal creating a clear image. In (B), there is an increased angle of incidence resulting in less clarity (anisotropic artifact). In (C), the angle of incidence is much greater resulting in more extreme anisotropic artifact with darkening of the structures.

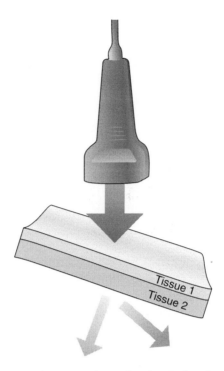

FIGURE 2.9 Illustration demonstrating refraction. Refraction is the alteration of direction of the sound wave after it strikes the interface of different tissue with different impedances. If the sound wave propagation velocity is faster in the first tissue (less impedance in tissue 1) then the refraction occurs toward the center (perpendicular to the interface) (green arrow). If the velocity is greater in the second tissue (less impedance in tissue 2) then the refraction is away from the incident beam (purple arrow).

Absorption

Another source of attenuation of the propagating sound wave is through *absorption*. This occurs when the sound wave energy is given off as heat. As a result, none of this energy returns to the transducer to contribute to the creation of the signal.

Scatter

Scatter refers to the propagation of incident sound waves in oblique directions. This occurs when the tissue being observed is not completely heterogeneous or has rough edges (Figure 2.10). The return of these obliquely propagated sound waves is termed *backscatter*. The random image pattern created by backscatter is termed *speckle*.

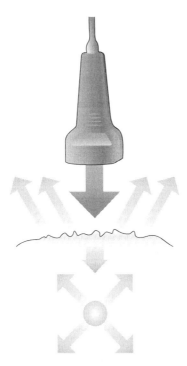

FIGURE 2.10 Illustration demonstrating principles of scatter. Scatter occurs when the incident sound wave (large red arrow) strikes on irregular or nonhomogeneous surface. Portions of the sound waves are scattered randomly, whereas the remainder continues on as a propagating wave (small red arrow). Scatter can also occur when the propagating wave strikes a smaller object such as a red blood cell.

Harmonic Frequency

Because of the varying characteristics and properties of tissue, ultrasonic waves can be produced which are not entirely linear. The return of this non-linear propagation to the transducers produces a pattern distinct from the more linear return echo. These waves are called *harmonic frequency* waves. These waves are of generally higher frequency than the original sound waves. In some circumstances, the harmonic frequency waves can be evaluated and it can provide an image that has fewer artifacts than the primary propagated wave. This is particularly useful with tissue that has significantly contrasting density.

TISSUE PROPERTIES

Speed of Sound Waves

The speed of sound wave transmission is affected by the properties of the medium in which it is traveling. Sound waves generally travel more slowly in gas mediums, faster in fluids, and fastest in solid material. Ultrasound waves travel through most human tissue at a speed of 1,540 m/s. Ultrasound instruments use this speed for timing the returning echoes to calculate the depth of tissue and constructing images.

Acoustic Impedance

Acoustic impedance refers to a tissue's property that allows propagation of sound waves. Higher acoustic impedance of the tissue results in less propagation of the sound wave. The amount of the sound energy reflected back to the transducer is directly proportional to the difference in acoustic impedance between tissues. Tissue interfaces with a larger difference in acoustic impedance will result in a larger amount of sound energy reflected back to the transducer. This results in the production of a brighter (hyperechoic) signal. An example of this is muscle tissue with relatively low acoustic impedance, next to bone tissue with very high acoustic impedance. The resultant reflection from this interface produces a very bright (hyperechoic) signal (Figure 2.11).

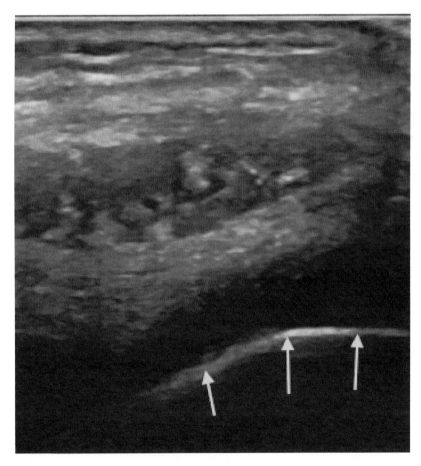

FIGURE 2.11 Sonogram demonstrating the bright signal characteristics from a location with a large difference in tissue impedance. The hyperechoic (bright) signal is seen with relatively low-impedance tissue next to high-impedance bone.

· ·

1) High-frequency sound waves help provide higher resolution images of relatively superficial structures but low-frequency sound waves have better penetration of deeper tissue.
2) Keep the incident sound waves as close to perpendicular to the tissue under evaluation as possible to allow most of the sound waves to return back to the transducer and therefore, produce best visualization.
3) Reflection of sound waves back from the tissues with the largest difference in impedance provides the most hyperechoic (brightest) signals. Bone has a very high impedance and appears hyperechoic on ultrasound.

BIBLIOGRAPHY

1. Connolly D, Berman L, McNally E. The use of beam angulation to overcome anisotropy when viewing human tendon with high frequency linear array ultrasound. *Br J Radiol*. 2001;74:183-185.

2. Entrekin RR, Porter BA, Sillesen HH, et al. Real-time spatial compound imaging: application to breast, vascular, and musculoskeletal ultrasound. *Semin Ultrasound CT MR*. 2001;22(1):50-64.

3. Kremkau FW. *Diagnostic Ultrasound: Principles and Ultrasound*. St. Louis, MO: Saunders; 2002.

3

Understanding the Equipment

The vast array of controls on most ultrasound machines can create anxiety for the beginner. Developing an understanding of the purpose of the instrumentation will facilitate the ability to create an optimal image of the tissue intended. Although daunting to some at first glance, systematically learning the purpose and utility of the controls can be accomplished easily in a relatively short amount of time.

TRANSDUCERS

The transducer is often considered the most important component of the ultrasound machine (Figure 3.1). The characteristics of the transducer determine much of the frequency and resolution of the image. The transducer contains a crystal matrix, typically quartz. It uses the reverse piezoelectric effect described in Chapter 2, to create sound waves that enter the tissue of interest, which are then reflected back. The transducer receives the reflected sound waves and converts them into electrical impulses (piezoelectric effect) used to create the ultrasound image. During active scanning, the transducer typically receives sound waves 80% of the time and transmits sound waves during the other 20%.

There are different types of transducers used in ultrasound.

The traditional transducer types utilized for high-frequency musculoskeletal ultrasound include linear, curvilinear, and small footprint or *hockey stick* (Figure 3.2). Linear transducers are used for most

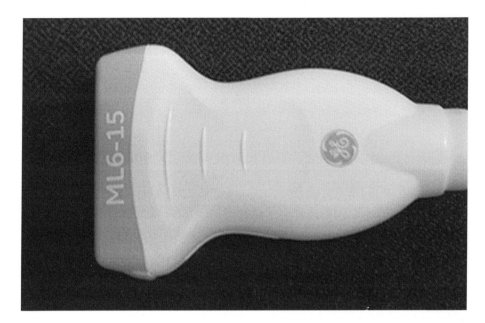

FIGURE 3.1 Picture of a linear broadband transducer.

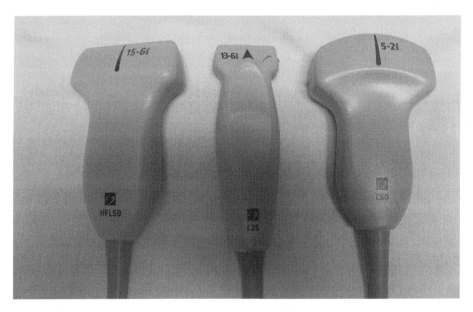

FIGURE 3.2 Picture of different types of transducers typically used for musculoskeletal ultrasound evaluations. From left to right, there is a linear, small footprint, and curvilinear transducer.

musculoskeletal applications. They are generally high-frequency broadband transducers that are designed to provide high-resolution images of relatively superficial structures (Figure 3.3). By contrast, curvilinear transducers should be used when images of deeper structures are needed, such as the hip. In general, the higher frequency linear transducers should be used whenever

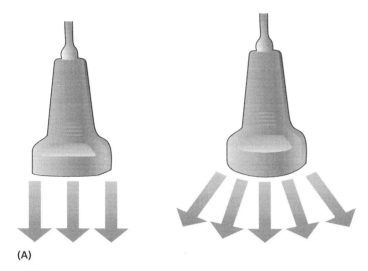

(A)

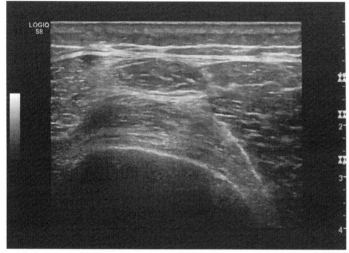

(B)

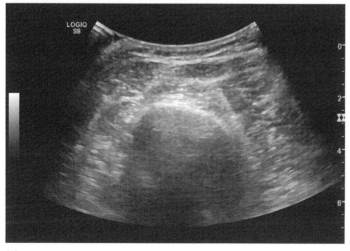

(C)

FIGURE 3.3 Demonstration of differences between a linear and curvilinear transducer. (A) An illustration of beam direction emitted from a linear (left) transducer versus a curvilinear (right). Note that the beam direction emitted from a curvilinear transducer extends to a wider area. It also emits lower frequency sound waves that extend deeper. The profile of the higher frequency linear transducer provides better resolution for more superficial structures. (B) Sonogram showing the appearance of the image created by a linear transducer. (C) Sonogram showing the appearance of the image created by a curvilinear transducer.

possible to provide the best image. The small footprint transducers are linear transducers that are sometimes desirable when imaging around smaller areas or bony prominences.

In some clinical situations, it can be advantageous to use more than one type of transducer. An example would be screening a larger field with a curvilinear transducer, and then subsequently focusing on a smaller region with a linear transducer for greater detail. The examiner should not hesitate to switch transducers if the optimal image is not initially obtained and different depth or frequency is needed.

ULTRASOUND IMAGING MODES

There are different echo display modes used by ultrasound machines. This includes A-mode (amplitude), B-mode (brightness), and M-mode (motion).

A-mode provides a display of the processed information versus time. It is the simplest form of ultrasound. A single transducer scans a line through the body and the images plotted are a function of depth of the tissue. Currently, A-mode is rarely used for medical diagnostic ultrasound, with the exception of some ophthalmology applications.

B-mode uses A-mode information and converts it into dots that are modulated by brightness (Figure 3.4). B-mode is also known as *2D-mode*

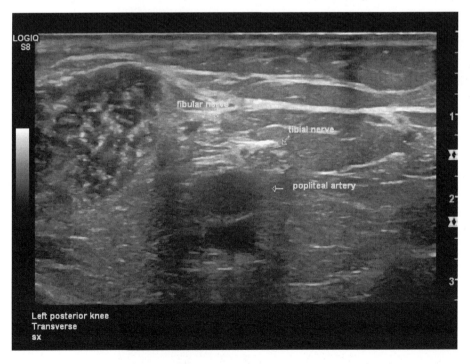

FIGURE 3.4 Sonogram showing the characteristic gray scale image of B-mode (2D) ultrasound.

and uses a linear array of transducers to create a two-dimensional (2D) image of a plane of tissue. This is the imaging mode used in most medical ultrasound applications and currently almost exclusively in musculoskeletal sonography. The basic physics of the creation of the B-mode image is discussed in Chapter 2.

M-mode uses B-mode information and displays the echoes from a moving organ. Ultrasound pulses are emitted in quick succession and the reflections from the moving organ provide information on the position of its boundaries. This is roughly analogous to recording an ultrasound movie (Figure 3.5).

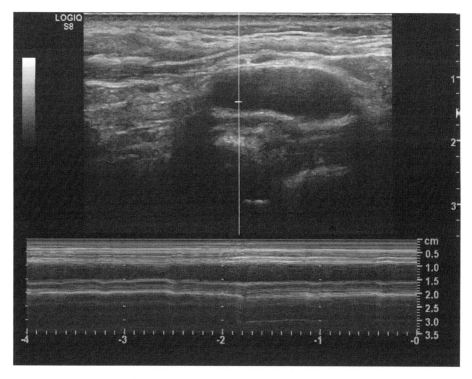

FIGURE 3.5 Sonogram showing M-mode ultrasound. This mode captures the returning echoes in only a single line of the B-mode image and displays them over time. In this sonogram, the B-mode (top) and M-mode (bottom) images are displayed in the same view on the screen.

DEPTH

The depth control changes the size of the area imaged. The goal of selecting the appropriate depth setting is to see deep enough into the field desired, but also limit wasted space below the image. An excessively deep setting minimizes the size of the structures desired (Figure 3.6). Most machines have depth measurement on the screen (Figure 3.7). This facilitates measurement of the structure size and depth of the field.

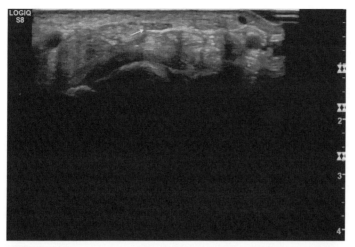

(A)

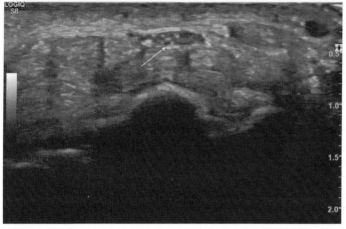

(B)

FIGURE 3.6 Sonograms demonstrating the proper use of the depth setting. (A) Demonstrates an image with excessive depth resulting in significant wasted space and more difficulty seeing the desired structure (median nerve—yellow arrow). (B) Demonstrates a more appropriate use of the depth setting to provide a better image of the structure of interest.

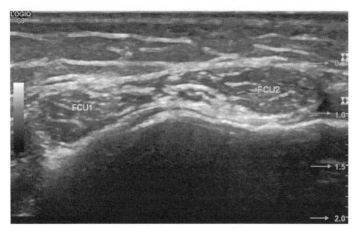

FIGURE 3.7 Sonogram showing the depth scale to the right of the screen (in yellow, illuminated by the blue arrows). This scale is labeled in centimeters with each mark representing 1 mm. The depth of this entire image is 2 cm.

FREQUENCY CONTROL

The frequency control determines the frequency of the sound wave emission from the broadband transducer. As discussed in Chapter 2, the higher frequencies provide better resolution for superficial structures, but do not penetrate to deeper tissue as well as lower frequencies (Figure 2.3). It is common to change the frequency setting repeatedly during an ultrasound evaluation to optimize visualization of both deep and superficial structures.

GRAY SCALE GAIN

The gray scale gain essentially controls the brightness of the image. It is analogous to the volume knob on a radio. It is increased if a brighter image is desired and decreased if a darker image is desired (Figure 3.8). Changing the gain does not affect the resolution but can often provide variations in contrast between different types of tissues.

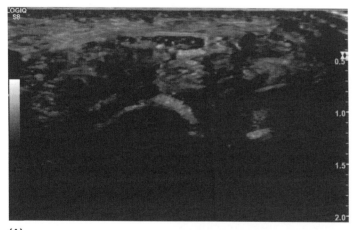

(A)

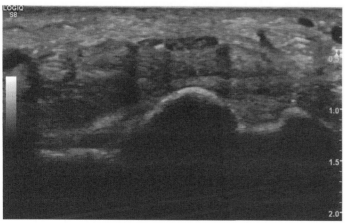

FIGURE 3.8 Sonogram of a short-axis view of the median nerve and surrounding flexor tendons with progressively higher gain. The image in (A) has the lowest gain and is darkest. The image in (C) has the higher gain and is the brightest of the three.

(B)

(continued)

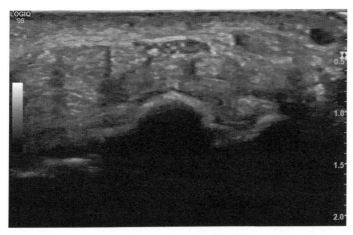

(C)

FIGURE 3.8 (*continued*)

TIME GAIN COMPENSATION

The time gain compensation (TGC) is often the most intimidating control on the ultrasound machine for beginners (Figure 3.9). Despite the multiple knobs, it is simply a control to allow segmental gain changes from top to bottom of the image (Figure 3.10). With the instrument shown, when the control is moved toward the right, that corresponding segment becomes brighter. Conversely when the control is moved to the left, its corresponding segment of the image becomes darker. All of the controls are generally kept close to the middle for most scanning purposes. The controls are moved when there is a desire to emphasize or de-emphasize a certain level or levels of the image.

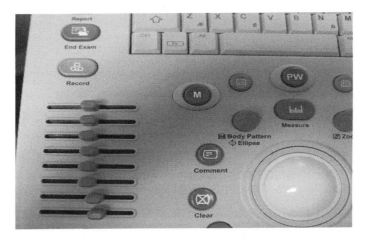

FIGURE 3.9 Picture of the TGC controls (lower left portion of the picture) on the ultrasound machine.

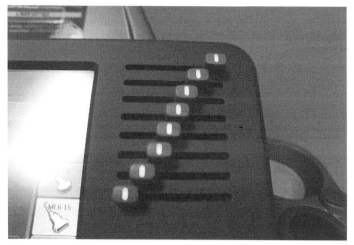

(A)

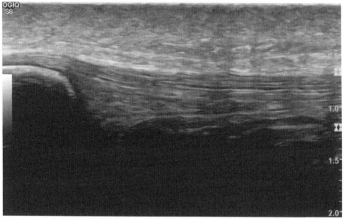

(B)

FIGURE 3.10 Picture of the TGC control configuration and the corresponding result of the sonogram appearance. The gain control for each control knob corresponds to its relative position on the screen. For example, the control knob at the top alters the gain for the top segment of the image and the control knob at the bottom alters the gain for the bottom segment of the image. The control settings positioned as in picture (A) creates an image as in (B) with the top segment the brightest, the middle segment moderately bright, and the lower segment the darkest. Reversing the control settings (C) makes the top segment the darkest and the bottom the brightest (D). Moving all of the TGC controls to the left (E) creates the darkest image based on the gain settings (F). Moving all of the TGC controls to the right (G) creates the brightest image (H). Placing the TGC controls to the middle (I) creates a uniform gain (J). Note that the darker appearance in the deeper aspect of the image in (J) is mostly a reflection of the depth of tissue and that level and the relative penetration of the incident sound waves.

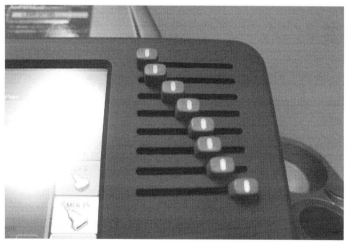

(C)

(continued)

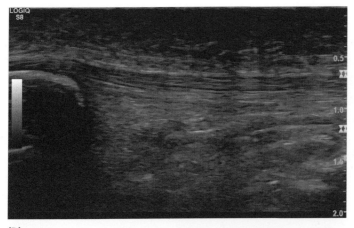

(D)

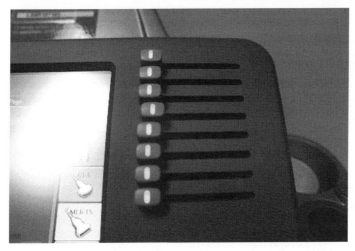

(E)

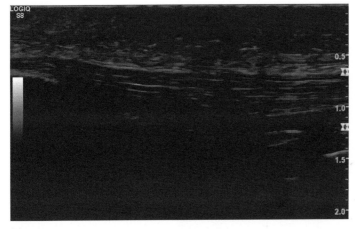

(F)

FIGURE 3.10 *(continued)*

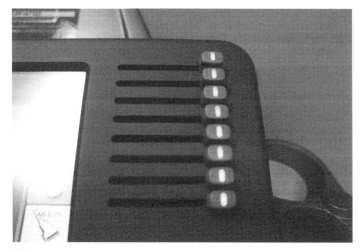

(G)

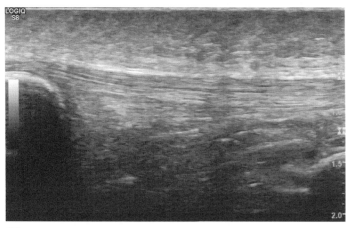

(H)

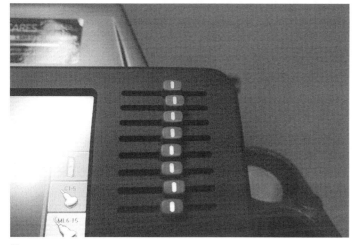

(I)

FIGURE 3.10 (*continued*)

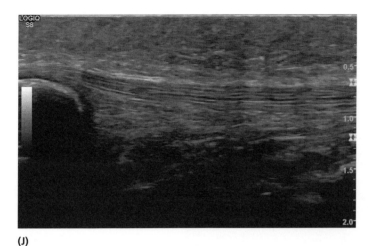

(J)

FIGURE 3.10 (continued)

MAPPING

Mapping is used to create differences in image color and contrast. Some of the mapping changes can be relatively subtle and the appearance of the image is often merely personal preference (Figure 3.11). For most common musculoskeletal examinations, frequent mapping changes are unnecessary. It is reasonable to become familiar with different mapping effects on the image as scanning skills progress. Changing the *tint* can also influence the appearance and color of the image (Figure 3.12). These changes are also personal preference and are less commonly utilized in routine musculoskeletal evaluations.

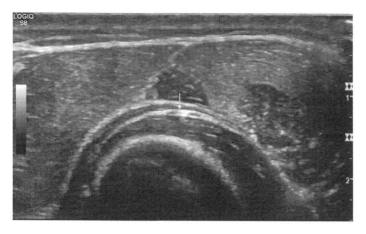

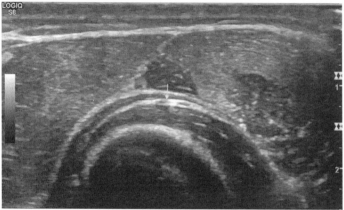

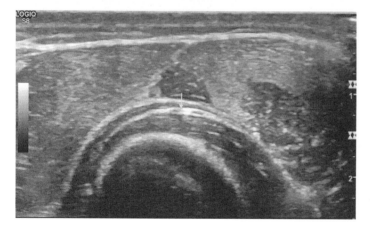

FIGURE 3.11 Sonograms of the same structure with different mapping. Some of the differences are relatively subtle and mapping is often personal preference; however, mapping can be used to provide improved discrimination between tissues. In this image, mapping changes can help provide better conspicuity of the deep branch of the radial nerve (yellow arrow).

(*continued*)

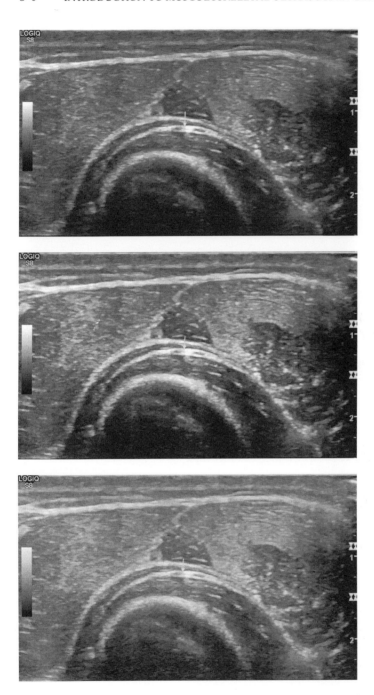

FIGURE 3.11 (*continued*)

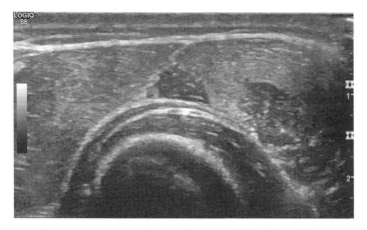

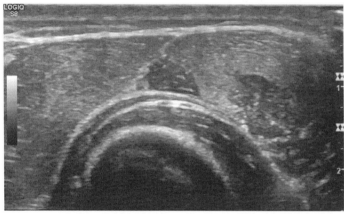

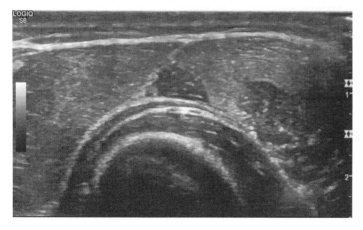

FIGURE 3.12 Sonograms of the same structure shown in Figure 3.11 but with different tints.

(*continued*)

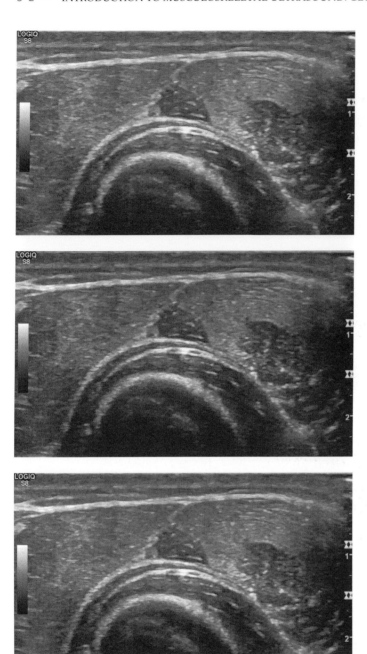

FIGURE 3.12 (continued)

DOPPLER IMAGING

Both color and power Doppler controls are a vital part of musculoskeletal ultrasound scanning. Their application and clinical utility are discussed in more detail in Chapter 6. Doppler imaging detects movement and therefore, is useful for detecting blood flow. Power Doppler is highly sensitive for movement and is depicted by red (or orange) hue (Figure 3.13). Color Doppler detects direction of flow in relation to the transducer and is depicted by red (toward the transducer) and blue (away from the transducer) colors (Figure 3.14).

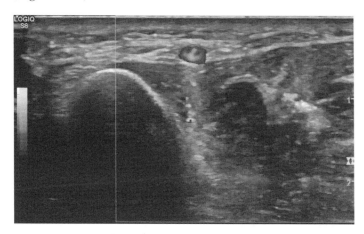

FIGURE 3.13 Sonogram using power Doppler to demonstrate flow through the radial artery in short axis. Note that the flow in power Doppler is depicted exclusively in red.

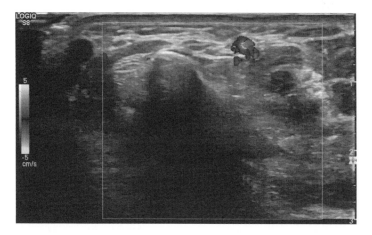

FIGURE 3.14 Sonogram using color Doppler to demonstrate flow through the radial artery in short axis. Note that the flow can be depicted in either red (toward the transducer) or blue (away from the transducer) or both.

SPLIT SCREEN

Many ultrasound machines allow simultaneous images to be produced on the video console. This feature can provide simultaneous visualization of side-to-side comparison images (Figure 3.15). It can also be used to juxtapose sequential images to create a smoother single image over a larger field when slight position changes of the transducer is needed to produce clarity (Figure 3.16).

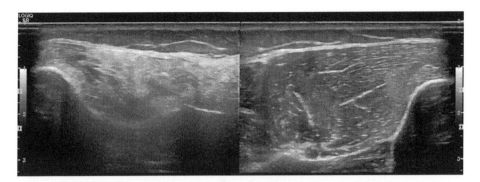

FIGURE 3.15 Sonogram demonstrating the value of using a split-screen image for side-to-side comparisons. In this instance, anterior compartment muscle in the leg with neurogenic atrophy (image on left) is compared with the normal leg at the same position (image on the right).

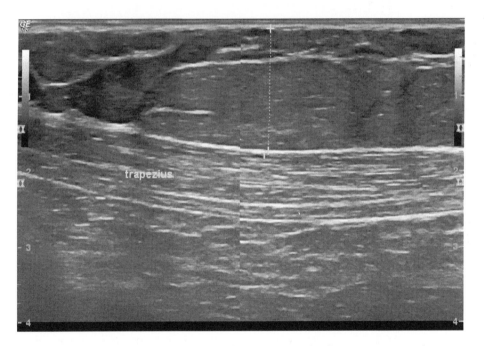

FIGURE 3.16 Sonogram showing the use of the juxtaposed split screen to extend the view of a longer image (in this example, trapezius and overlying lipoma) in long-axis view.

MARKING AND MEASUREMENT TOOL

Ultrasound machines have capabilities of very precise tissue measurement. The examiner should be familiar with controls for measurement. Most machines have the capability to perform multiple linear measurements, as well as to trace circular structures for cross-sectional area (Figure 3.17).

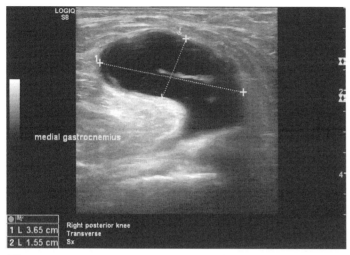

(A)

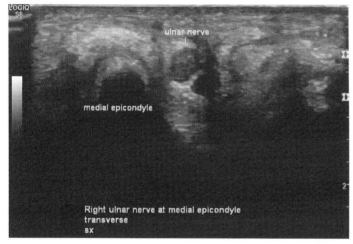

(B)

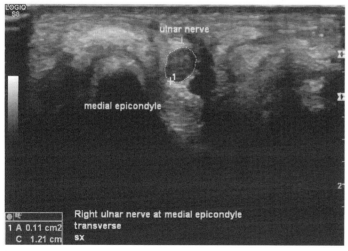

(C)

FIGURE 3.17 Sonograms demonstrating the use of measurement tools with ultrasound. The image in (A) shows the use of linear measurement of a Baker's cyst. The length in centimeters is shown in the left lower corner. The image in (B) shows the ulnar nerve in short axis at the level of the ulnar groove. The image in (C) shows the postmeasurement view. The cross-sectional area (A) of the nerve is shown in centimeters squared, the circumference (C) is shown in centimeters.

LABELING

Detailed image labeling is helpful for communication of results as well as future reference. It is important to identify the right or left side of the body as well as the orientation of the structure being imaged. The pertinent structure should be named as well as its orientation. Markers such as arrows are generally available to indicate the focal area of interest. When side-to-side images are being used, it is often helpful to label the symptomatic and asymptomatic side for clarity for the observer (Figure 3.18).

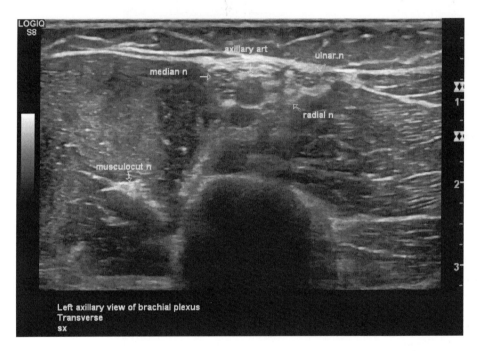

FIGURE 3.18 Sonogram demonstrating the use of labeling for orientation. In this example, the terminal branch level of the brachial plexus is shown. The structures of interest are identified. The side and area of the body are labeled. The view (transverse) is labeled and there is mention that this is the symptomatic side (sx) in the event there are left-to-right comparisons. The purpose of the detailed labeling is to allow review of the images and facilitate the correct orientation and identification for other observers.

IMAGE STORAGE

Image storage is needed to allow the pictures to be viewed at a later time. Printers are usually available with most machines and many can burn DVDs to allow the cinematography images to be carried to other locations, including physician appointments (Figure 3.19). Most machines have substantial data storage to allow the images to be viewed at a later time. The use of external hard drives for additional storage will help prevent the ultrasound machine from running out of memory.

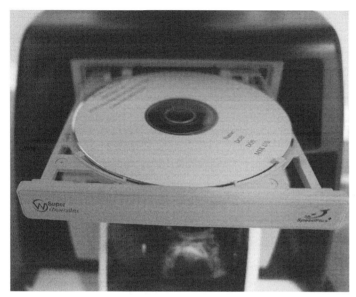

(A)

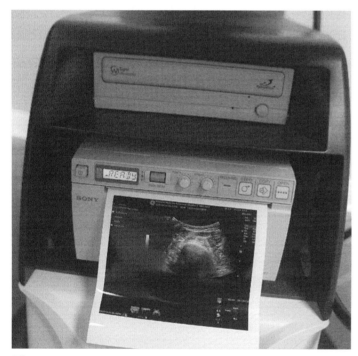

(B)

FIGURE 3.19 Pictures demonstrating examples of devices used for image storage and display. (A) DVD burner. (B) Printer for paper images. The printers allow easy viewing of the images. The DVDs can be transferred easily to other offices and include the motions loops.

GEL AND STANDOFF PADS

Ultrasound requires a solid medium to transmit a signal and provide a clear picture. Most frequently conduction gel or standoff pads are used for this purpose. Liberal use of this medium can prevent distortion of the image (Figure 3.20).

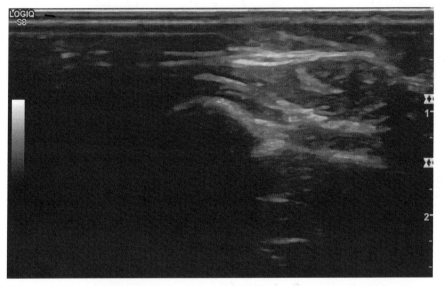

(A)

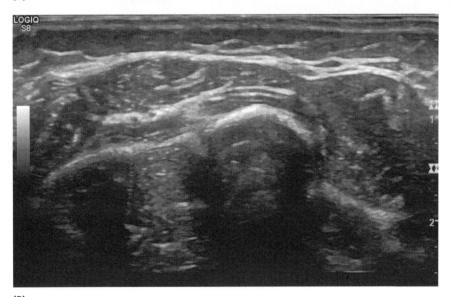

(B)

FIGURE 3.20 Sonograms demonstrating the value of adequate medium (gel) between the transducer and the skin of the patient. (A) Image with insufficient transmission gel and resultant poor quality. (B) Image of the same body region (forearm) with adequate gel eliminating the artifact from incomplete sound transmission back to the transducer with greatly improved quality.

CLEANING THE INSTRUMENT

The ultrasound transducer is the portion of the machine that makes contact with the patient and should be cleaned after each application. The transducer should be cleaned with soap and water or with low-level disinfectants such as quaternary ammonium sprays or wipes. Alcohol has the potential to damage the crystals in the transducer and should be avoided. The transducer should then be dried completely with a soft towel or cloth. Routine cleaning should not be confused with high-level disinfection required of internal and intraoperative probes. Protocols for higher level disinfection frequently change. In the United States, the Centers for Disease Control and Prevention website can be used for a reference.

ADVANCED CONTROLS

Some machines come with more advanced controls that include beam steering to change the angle of the incident sound waves emitted from the transducer, extended field of view to allow imaging over longer structures, and three-dimensional imaging among others. Detailed discussion of these and other advanced features are beyond the scope of this introductory text. Eventual mastery of these techniques will provide even greater imaging capabilities in the future.

REMEMBER ···

1) Take the time to learn the instrumentation in detail to develop the highest quality scanning.
2) Select the appropriate broadband transducer for the tissue being scanned. Generally, the highest frequency available that can adequately reach the tissue is desired.
3) When first learning your way around the machine, use the B-mode button to return to the basic 2D scanning mode.

BIBLIOGRAPHY

1. Centers for Disease Control and Prevention. *Guideline for Disinfection and Sterilization in Healthcare Facilities, 2008.* Atlanta, GA: Centers for Disease Control and Prevention website; 2008. http://www.cdc.gov/hicpac/pdf/guidelines/Disinfection_Nov_2008.pdf.

2. Koibuchi H, Fujii Y, Kotani K, et al. Degradation of ultrasound probes caused by disinfection with alcohol. *J Med Ultrasonics.* 2011;38:97–100.

3. Mirza WA, Imam SH, Kharal MS, et al. Cleaning methods for ultrasound probes. *J Coll Physicians Surg Pak.* 2008;18:286–289.

4. Nielsen TJ, Lambert MJ. Physics and instrumentation. In: Ma OJ, Mateer JR, eds. *Emergency Ultrasound.* New York, NY: McGraw-Hill; 2003:45–46.

5. Smith RS, Fry WR. Ultrasound instrumentation. *Surg Clin North Am.* 2004;84:953–971.

Image Optimization

Once the instrumentation has been reasonably mastered, the examiner can then strive to optimize the image desired. The goal is to have the image centered with sufficient clarity and the best resolution possible. The desired image should fill the majority of the screen. The settings should provide the optimal contrast between the tissues being examined. Appropriate labels and markings should also be added for future reference and for recognition by outside observers. Not all ultrasound machines are designed the same and some have frequencies, focal zones, and gray scale mapping that are already determined. Most machines have "pre-sets" with appropriate settings already determined for the type of tissue being scanned. Despite this, the examiner should have an understanding of the various components of ultrasonography to optimize the image in different circumstances.

ORIENT THE IMAGE

The image should be oriented in a reasonably consistent fashion. By convention, when a structure is imaged in long-axis plane, it is typically oriented so that the left of the screen is cranial and the right of the screen is caudal (Figure 4.1). There is generally less convention with respect to imaging structures in short axis. Some maintain the left of the screen as the anatomic right and others orient the left of the screen as the medial aspect of the body. It is probably best to perform short-axis live scanning in a position that makes sense with the orientation of the patient with respect to the screen. For example, when the transducer moves in the medial direction on the body, it should move the same direction on the screen (Figure 4.2).

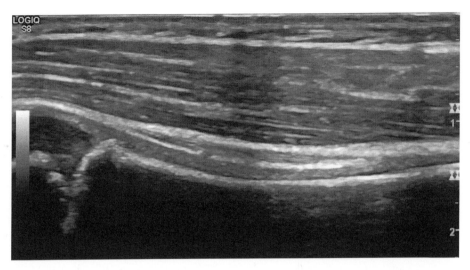

FIGURE 4.1 Sonogram of a long-axis view of the long head of the biceps brachii tendon. The image is oriented so that the left portion of the screen is toward the head.

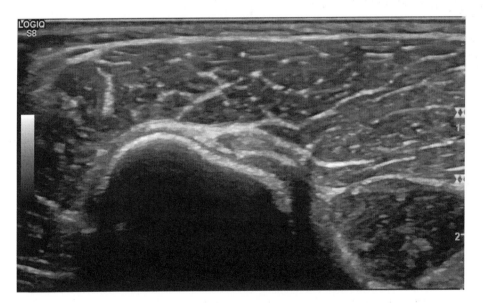

FIGURE 4.2 Sonogram of a short-axis view of the biceps brachii tendon shown in Figure 4.1. The left portion of the screen corresponds to the anatomic right (lateral) of the patient.

CENTERING THE IMAGE WITH THE TRANSDUCER

The image should be centered in the screen and maintained in that position during live scanning (Figure 4.3). This transducer skill should be practiced when first starting to scan. It is needed to prevent the desired image from repeatedly drifting out of view when scanning more rapidly.

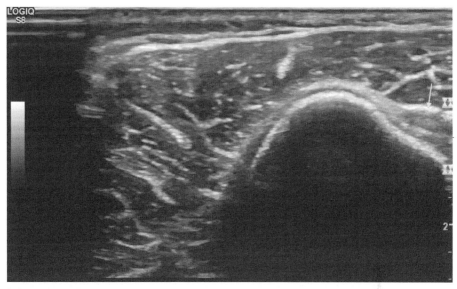

(A)

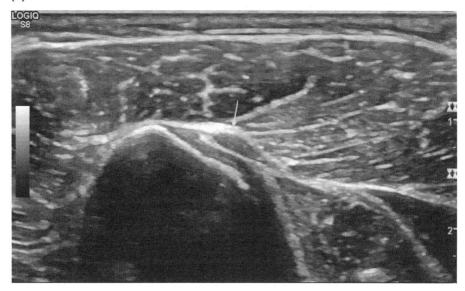

(B)

FIGURE 4.3 Sonograms demonstrating proper centering of the image. The image in (A) shows the structure of interest (yellow arrow) too far to the right in the picture. The image in (B) shows proper placement of the structure of interest in the center.

SELECT THE APPROPRIATE DEPTH

The depth should be set at the level that places the desired tissue in the majority of the screen. Too much depth results in the desired image appearing too small with essentially wasted space. If the depth is too low, the desired image could be truncated or there can simply be insufficient contrast from surrounding tissue to provide adequate perspective (Figure 4.4).

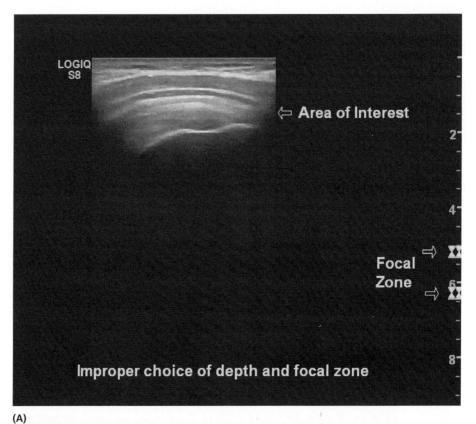

(A)

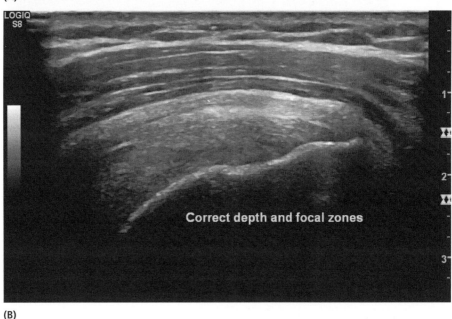

(B)

FIGURE 4.4 Sonograms demonstrating improper and proper depth setting and use of focal zones. In (A), the setting is too deep for the image desired resulting in wasted space and decreased visualization if the pertinent structures. The focal zones are also set improperly diminishing the resolution of the structure (supraspinatus tendon) intended. The image in (B) demonstrates appropriate setting of the depth and focal zones for image optimization.

SELECT THE APPROPRIATE FREQUENCY

As described in Chapter 3, higher frequencies are used for resolution of more superficial structures and lower frequencies are used for better tissue penetration. There are no hard and fast rules regarding the precise frequency for each specific depth as it can vary due to a number of factors including tissue thickness. A general rule is that the highest frequency that provides adequate tissue penetration should be utilized (Figure 4.5).

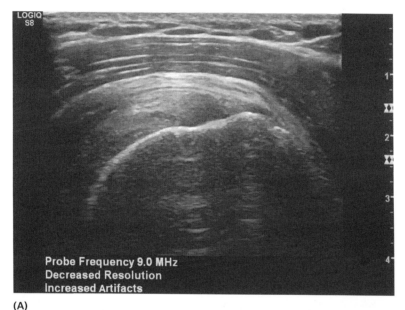

(A)

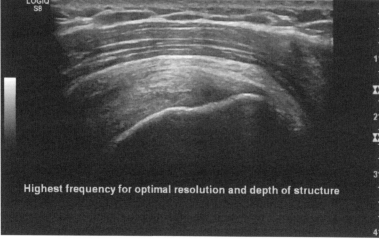

(B)

FIGURE 4.5 Sonograms demonstrating the effect of frequency on the image. In (A), the frequency is set too low (9 MHz) for the relatively superficial structure (supraspinatus tendon) resulting in an unnecessary artifact. In (B), the appropriate frequency (15 MHz) provides a clearer image of the tendon with less artifact.

SELECT THE APPROPRIATE FOCAL ZONE

The focal zone is the horizontal line on the screen that should be placed at the level of greatest interest on the screen. The focal zone refers to the location where the ultrasound beams converge to provide the greatest level of clarity (Figure 4.6). Failure to maintain the focal zone in the proper location with scanning will result in decreased resolution at the point desired (Figure 4.4). More than one focal zone can be used if the area of interest is larger than the single horizontal level; however, additional focal zones tend to decrease the frame rate. The frame rate refers to the speed in which the image regains clarity after the transducer is moved. For this reason, too many focal zones make the image harder to see when the transducer is moved rapidly.

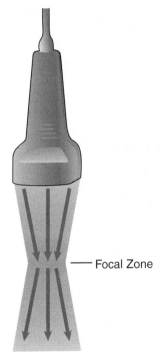

— Focal Zone

FIGURE 4.6 Illustration demonstrating the focal zone of the ultrasound beam. This is the region where the majority of the incident sound waves converge to create the greatest degree of clarity.

SELECT THE APPROPRIATE GAIN

The gain increases or decreases the brightness of the image. The gain is typically set to provide the right contrast between the tissues being observed. This is often a matter of preference but extremes of high or low gain should generally be avoided (Figure 3.8).

SELECT THE GRAY SCALE MAPPING WHEN NEEDED

The gray scale mapping can be utilized to provide the desired color to the picture. This is often merely personal preference, but the mapping should be used that gives the optimal contrast between the tissues of interest (Figure 3.11).

MINIMIZE ANISOTROPIC ARTIFACT

Anisotropic artifact is discussed in more detail in Chapter 13. This artifact occurs when the incident sound waves are not orthogonal to the desired structures resulting in less return of the waves to the transducer and resultant decreased clarity of the image (Figure 4.7).

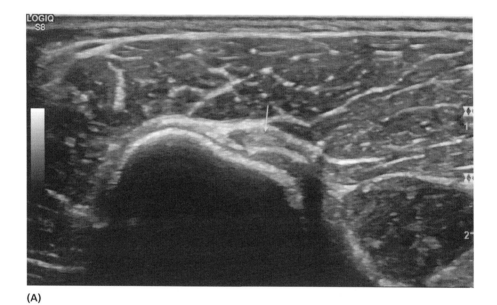

(A)

FIGURE 4.7 Sonograms demonstrating the effect of anisotropy on a biceps brachii tendon in short axis. In image (A), the incident beam has an angle of incidence that is greater than 0°, or less than perpendicular in relation to the tendon (yellow arrow).

(continued)

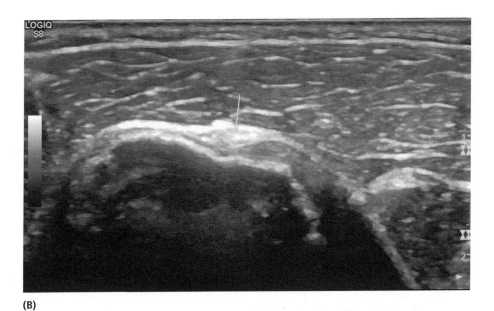

(B)

FIGURE 4.7 (*continued*) Note the more hyperechoic (brighter) signal intensity of the tendon when the incident beam is placed in a perpendicular position in relation to the tendon in (B).

ADD THE APPROPRIATE LABELS

The labels should readily identify the structures being evaluated in the picture and include the orientation and side of the body. In side-to-side comparison imaging, it is often appropriate to clarify the symptomatic side. Arrows to indicate specific areas of attention and measurement tools should also be placed when needed. The labels should be easy to read and positioned in a location that does not obstruct visualization of the desired image (Figure 3.18).

REMEMBER ··

1) Always have clear orientation to the position of the image. Structures in long axis by convention should have the cranial aspect toward the left of the screen and the caudal end toward the right of the screen.
2) Make sure the focal zone is placed at the level of the structure desired.
3) Orient the incident sound waves in an orthogonal (perpendicular) position to the tissue desired to minimize anisotropic artifact.

BIBLIOGRAPHY

1. Malanga G, Mautner K. *Atlas of Ultrasound-Guided Musculoskeletal Injections.* New York, NY: McGraw-Hill; 2013.

2. Smith J, Finnoff JT. Diagnostic and interventional musculoskeletal ultrasound: part 1. Fundamentals. *PM&R*. 2009;1(1):64–75.

3. Strakowski JA. *Ultrasound Evaluation of Focal Neuropathies. Correlation With Electrodiagnosis.* New York, NY: Demos Medical; 2014.

4. Van Holsbeeck MT, Introcaso JS. *Musculoskeletal Ultrasound.* 2nd ed. St. Louis, MO: Mosby; 2001.

5

Scanning Techniques and Ergonomics

INTRODUCTION

Development of proper positioning and scanning early on in training is paramount to success later on. The goal should be to have an arrangement in which both the patient and examiner are comfortable to make image acquisition easily and efficiently. Proper mechanics will help prevent fatigue, strain, and overuse injuries common to ultrasonographers. Attention should be given to the manner in which the transducer is held and moved. Both the patient and examiner should be placed in proper position in relation to the screen and controls.

USE OF THE TRANSDUCER

Successful scanning requires an effective grip on the transducer. Novice scanners tend to hold the transducer inappropriately and with a grip that is too tight. The transducer should be held at the base to facilitate control (Figure 5.1). The grip should be firm without squeezing the transducer. In the same fashion as it is difficult to write well while gripping a pen too tightly, it is difficult to scan easily with good control while doing this with the transducer (Figure 5.2). It is also helpful to maintain contact with the patient while scanning to maintain stability and prevent the transducer from moving or rotating out of the image desired. Contacting the patient with the small and ring fingers and ulnar aspect of the hand while gripping the transducer with the thumb, index, and long fingers provides stability and optimizes scanning control. The examiner should also resist the urge to apply excessive pressure with the transducer as this can deform the image (Figure 5.3).

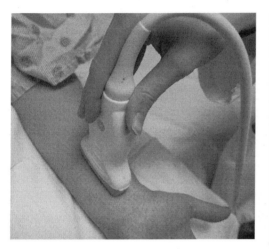
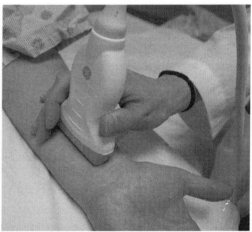

(A)   **(B)**

FIGURE 5.1 Pictures demonstrating the incorrect (A) and correct (B) methods of holding the transducer for optimal stability and control. In (A), the examiner is holding the transducer too far from the base and does not have contact with the patient. In the appropriate hand position in (B), the examiner has a comfortable grip of the transducer at its base with the thumb, index, and long fingers while maintaining good contact with the patient with the small and ring fingers and ulnar portion of the hand.

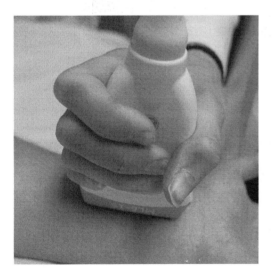
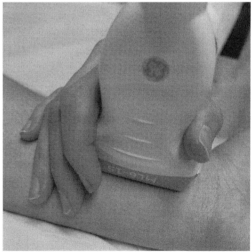

(A)   **(B)**

FIGURE 5.2 Pictures demonstrating excessive (A) and appropriate (B) grip when holding the transducer. In (A), the examiner is grasping the transducer with excessive grip resulting in more difficulty performing smooth transducer movements during the examination. Appropriate grip is shown in (B). This grip allows smooth and easy transducer movements with good balance and also does not create undue strain during the examination.

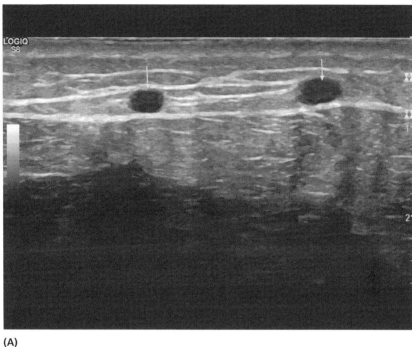

(A)

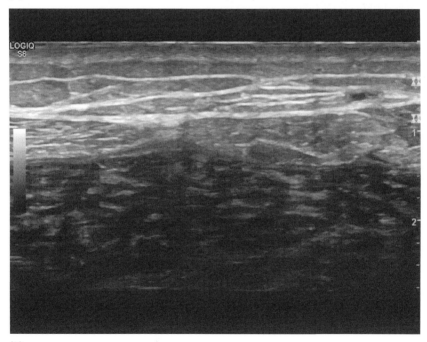

(B)

FIGURE 5.3 Sonograms demonstrating an example of the effect of increasing transducer pressure on the image. The image in (A) is performed with relatively minimal transducer pressure. Note the appearance of the veins (yellow arrows). In (B), the transducer pressure is increased. Note in that image, the transducer pressure has caused the veins to collapse and are no longer evident. In addition, the subcutaneous tissue at the top of the image is thinner than the image in (A). The examiner should always be vigilant about excessive pressure with the transducer, which can affect the appearance.

Plenty of conduction gel should be used for good contact and a clear image (Figure 3.20). Scanning is often performed with sweeping motions to visualize the area intended. In many circumstances, scanning more rapidly helps to distinguish different types of tissue and can improve conspicuity relative to the image created when scanning very slowly. Using back and forth scanning often will facilitate appreciation of different types of echotexture such as fascicular pattern of nerves compared to the fibrillar pattern of tendons.

The examiner should be comfortable using techniques to minimize anisotropic artifact. This includes changing the direction of the transducer beam to a more orthogonal (perpendicular) orientation of the tissue of interest when the angle of incidence is too small. Changing the direction of the beam by altering the angle without moving the base is called *toggling* the transducer (Figure 5.4). A *heel-to-toe* maneuver is used to improve the conspicuity of a curved structure in long axis (Figure 5.5). It is particularly effective in the circumstance of tendons in long axis that have a portion curved out of perpendicular orientation to the transducer (Figure 5.6).

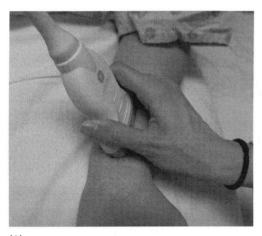 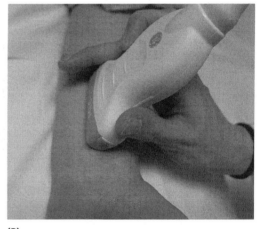

(A)   (B)

FIGURE 5.4 Pictures demonstrating toggling of the transducer to change the angle of incidence of the sound waves on the tissue. Note that the position angle of the transducer is changed from (A) to (B). This maneuver is used to reduce anisotropic artifact. The angle is changed without moving the base to a different position. Simultaneously moving the base while toggling should generally be avoided to prevent a confusing change of too many components of the image.

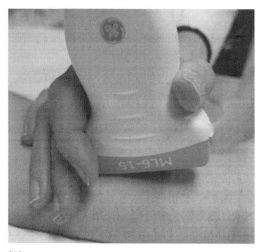 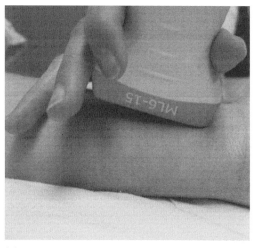

(A)   (B)

FIGURE 5.5 Pictures demonstrating the heel-to-toe rocking of the transducer to change the angle of incidence of the sound waves on the tissue. Note that the position of the transducer is changed from (A) to (B). This maneuver is used to reduce anisotropic artifact of tissue in long axis. With heel-to-toe rocking, the angle is changed without sliding the base to a different position.

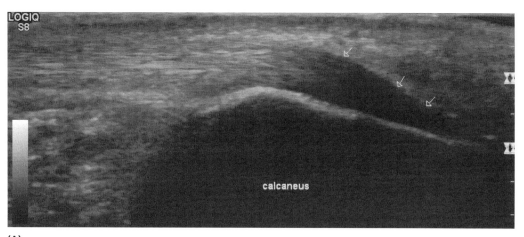

(A)

FIGURE 5.6 Sonograms demonstrating the effect of the heel-to-toe rocking maneuver on the appearance of the long-axis view of the Achilles tendon insertion at the calcaneus (yellow arrows). In (A), the incident sound waves have an increased angle of incidence with respect to the curved portion of the Achilles insertion. Note that the fibers appear hypoechoic (dark) in this location. In (B), the heel-to-toe rocking changes the beam to a more perpendicular orientation in relation to that area, reducing the hypoechoic anisotropic artifact. This maneuver helps distinguish this anisotropic artifact from pathologic change in the tendon fibers, which would persist in hypoechoic appearance despite the orientation change.

(continued)

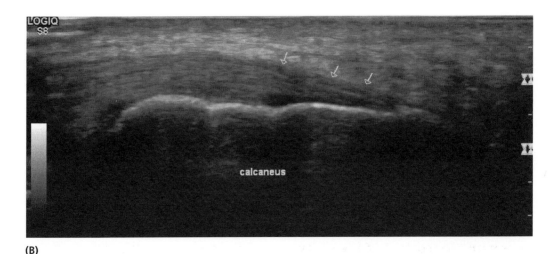

(B)

FIGURE 5.6 (*continued*)

ERGONOMICS

Attention to body position for both the examiner and the patient can improve the efficiency of the evaluation and minimize undue strain. The patient should be placed in a position that provides easy access with the transducer and allows comfortable arm position. Having to reach excessively can lead to fatigue and overuse syndromes (Figure 5.7). The patient should be generally placed between the examiner and the screen allowing visualization of both. This is important for both diagnostic evaluations as well as therapeutic injections (Figure 5.8). The machine should also be close enough to allow easy access to the controls without excessive moving. Attention to these details can make the scanning experience much easier for both the examiner and patient.

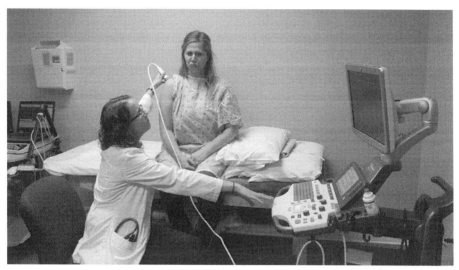

(A)

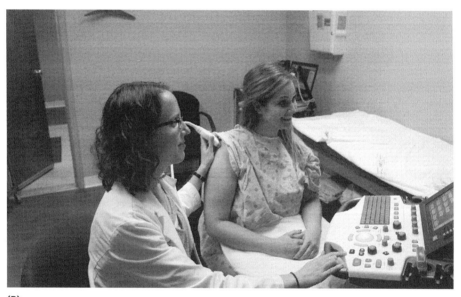

(B)

FIGURE 5.7 Pictures demonstrating poor (A) and good (B) positioning for performing an ultrasound evaluation. In the poor positioning (A), the examiner has to reach for the patient as well as the machine. This creates an inefficient examination with undue muscle strain and fatigue. The area being examined is not in line with the screen. In (B), note how both the patient and examiner are in comfortable positions. The examiner does not have to overextend to perform the scanning or reach the controls. The patient is relatively between the examiner and screen allowing the examiner to attend to both areas simultaneously. The patient is also able to see the screen during the examination, which can facilitate live demonstration and explanation of the findings.

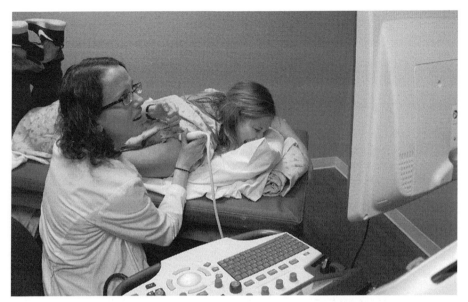

(A)

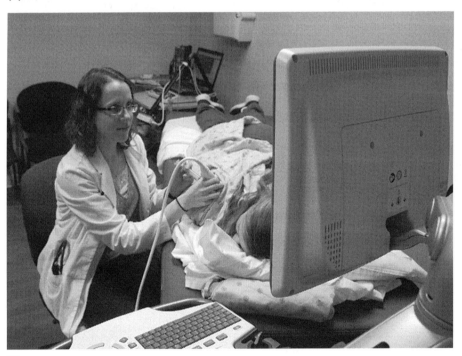

(B)

FIGURE 5.8 Pictures demonstrating poor (A) and good (B) positioning for performing an ultrasound-guided injection. In the poor positioning (A), the patient is in a position that is out of line with the screen. This results in the need to look away from the patient to see the screen and also difficult positioning. In (B), note how the patient is in between the practitioner performing the procedure and the machine. This facilitates visualization of both areas and easy access to the injection field and the controls of the machine.

REMEMBER ·

1) Avoid excessive grip and pressure with the transducer and hold it at its base.
2) Keep contact with the patient with the hand holding the transducer while scanning.
3) Learn the technique of toggling and heal-to-toe rocking with the transducer to reduce anisotropic artifact.
4) Use good ergonomics to provide a comfortable position for both the examiner and patient to improve ease of scanning.

BIBLIOGRAPHY

1. Malanga G, Mautner K. *Atlas of Ultrasound-Guided Musculoskeletal Injections*. New York, NY: McGraw-Hill; 2013.

2. Strakowski JA. *Ultrasound Evaluation of Focal Neuropathies. Correlation With Electrodiagnosis*. New York, NY: Demos Medical; 2014.

Doppler Imaging

Doppler imaging provides an important complement to the gray scale image in routine B-mode ultrasound. It provides color signal with movement, making it particularly useful for assessing vascular flow. Doppler imaging has a number of applications in musculoskeletal evaluations. It helps to identify certain vascular structures, gives an indication of vascular flow, and can also be used to assess for increased vascularity in pathologic conditions, as well as synovitis in rheumatologic diseases and other inflammatory conditions. It can be additionally used to assess for vascular clots, aneurysms, and anatomic variations. There are two conventional types used in musculoskeletal medicine, power and color Doppler.

POWER DOPPLER

Power Doppler encodes the power of the ultrasound signal rather than velocity and direction. It is sensitive for movement in any direction. It is a single color and appears red or red-orange (Figure 6.1).

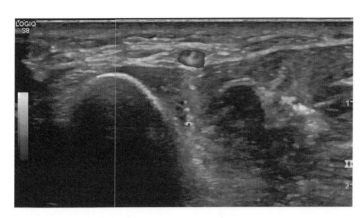

FIGURE 6.1 Sonogram demonstrating flow through the radial artery with power Doppler. The power Doppler signal reflects the power of the signal rather than the velocity or direction and is displayed in a single color (red).

COLOR DOPPLER

Color Doppler has both red and blue characteristics and provides information about directional movement. This is useful for determining the direction of vascular flow and is not to be confused with denoting venous or arterial blood. When the movement of the flow is toward the transducer, the Doppler is denoted in red. Blue is seen when the direction is away from the transducer (Figure 6.2).

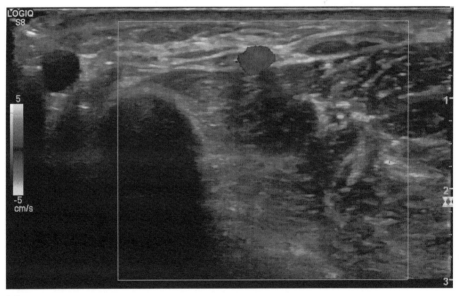

(A)

FIGURE 6.2 Sonograms demonstrating flow through the radial artery with color Doppler. The color Doppler signal is displayed in two colors (red and blue). The signal is more dependent on angle of the transducer with color Doppler. The different appearance of the same tissue in images (A)–(C) is related to changes in transducer position. The image in (A) appears similar to the power Doppler image in Figure 6.1. The transducer is oriented so that the flow is toward the transducer creating a red color. The image in (B) appears blue because the transducer is oriented so that the flow is away from the transducer. The image in (C) shows that the flow can have both colors when the transducer is oriented between the positions of (A) and (B).

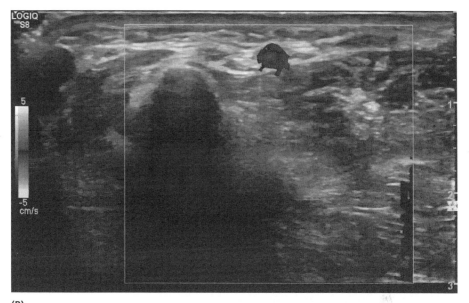

(B)

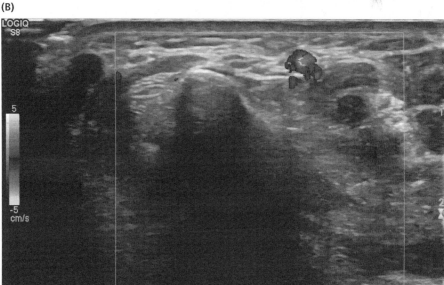

(C)

FIGURE 6.2 *(continued)*

COLOR VERSUS POWER DOPPLER

A weakness of color Doppler is that it can potentially miss flow that is perpendicular to the transducer. For this reason, it is useful to toggle the transducer to minimize that potential. Power Doppler signal is not dependent on direction, and it is more sensitive to movement than color Doppler, but its image can also be improved with toggling in some circumstances.

A disadvantage of the sensitivity of power Doppler to movement is that it is more likely to create flash artifact when the transducer or patient is

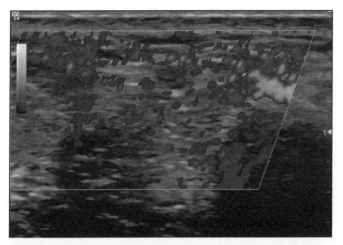

(A)

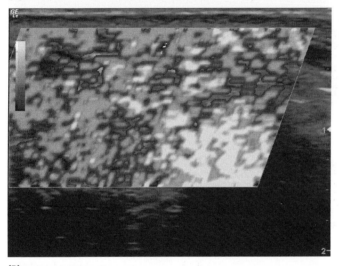

(B)

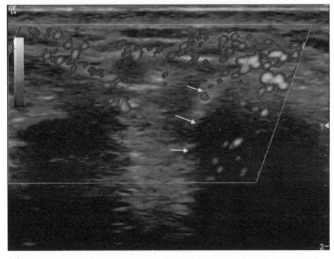

(C)

FIGURE 6.3 Sonograms demonstrating flash artifact with power Doppler due to transducer movement. The Doppler signal in images (A) and (B) is relatively easy to distinguish as artifact in light of the relatively massive extent. A clue that the signal is also artifact in (C) is the Doppler signal that is deep to the radial bony cortex (designated by the yellow arrows). True Doppler changes from vascularity cannot be seen through bone.

moving (Figure 6.3). By contrast, color Doppler is more likely than power Doppler to create artifact when the transducer is stationary. Both power and color Doppler have gain settings that affect their relative sensitivity. When the gain is set excessively high, there is an increase in artifact, even with the transducer and tissue at rest. If the gain is set too low, there is a loss of sensitivity. There remains a lack of standardization regarding appropriate gain settings for Doppler imaging, however, the gain should generally be set on the highest sensitivity that does not create significant artifact (Figure 6.4). One method used to establish the appropriate gain is to raise it initially, then gradually lower it to the point that no flow is seen beneath the cortex

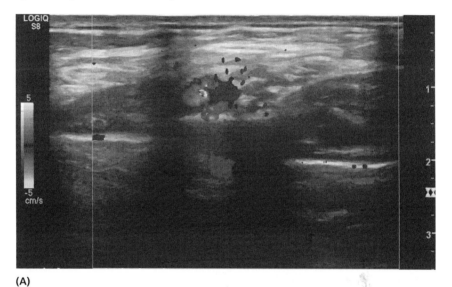

(A)

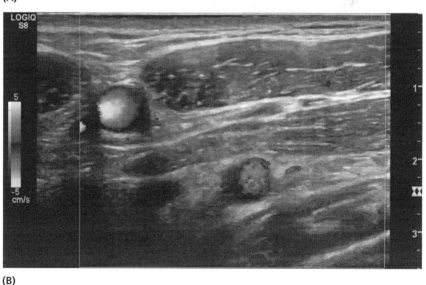

(B)

FIGURE 6.4 Sonograms demonstrating flash artifact with color Doppler. In (A), the gain is set somewhat high with an excessive amount of artifact seen extraneous to the vessel. The gain is set more appropriately in (B).

of bone. Sound waves do not readily penetrate bone, therefore Doppler flow seen below the cortex of bone should be considered artifact.

With nonvascular settings, color Doppler is preferable to power Doppler for assessment of high-flow vascular structures such as large arteries (Figure 6.5). Power Doppler is designed for low flow states and is therefore often preferable for smaller or deeper vessels and investigation for inflammation or neovascularization (Figure 6.6).

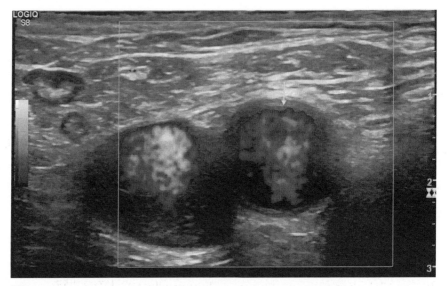

(A)

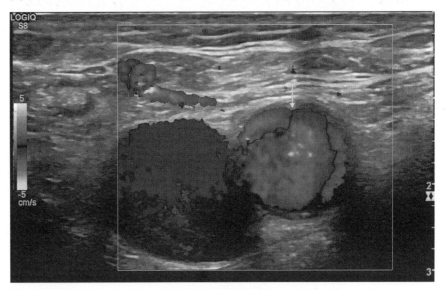

(B)

FIGURE 6.5 Sonograms demonstrating the appearance of both power (A) and color (B) Doppler of the femoral artery (yellow arrow). Note that the power Doppler signal does not completely fill the lumen of the artery, whereas the color Doppler signal does. Color Doppler is generally preferred for higher velocity flow states.

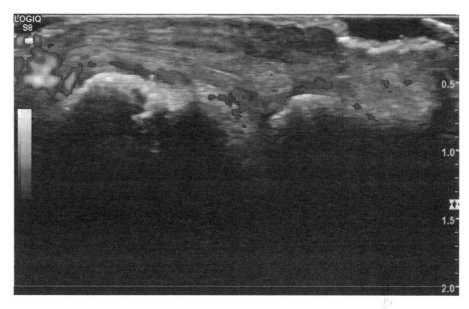

FIGURE 6.6 Sonogram demonstrating the use of power Doppler to show the effect of synovitis in the area of the metacarpal phalangeal joint in a patient with rheumatoid arthritis.

REMEMBER

1) Power Doppler is generally preferable for low flow states and color Doppler is used for higher flow states and assessment of direction.
2) Color Doppler has a two-color scale (red and blue) and assesses flow and direction. Red represents flow toward the transducer and blue represents flow away from the transducer.

BIBLIOGRAPHY

1. de Vos RJ, Weir A, Cobben LP, Tol JL. The value of power Doppler ultrasonography in Achilles tendinopathy: a prospective study. *Am J Sports Med*. 2007;35(10):1696–1701. Epub 2007 Jun 8.

2. Kremkau FW. *Diagnostic Ultrasound: Principles and Ultrasound*. St. Louis, MO: Saunders; 2002.

3. Nielsen TJ, Lambert MJ. Physics and instrumentation. In: MA OJ, Mateer JR, eds. *Emergency Ultrasound*. New York, NY: McGraw-Hill; 2003:45–46.

4. Rubin JM, Bude RO, Carson PL, et al. Power Doppler US: a potentially useful alternative to mean frequency-based color Doppler US. *Radiology*. 1994;190(3):853–856.

7

Imaging Tendon

Ultrasound is an excellent imaging modality for assessing tendons. Evaluation of tendon and tendonopathy is one of the most frequent uses of ultrasound in musculoskeletal medicine. Tendons are dynamic structures and highly visible with high-frequency ultrasound. Tendons are an important component of the musculoskeletal system by connecting muscle to bone.

TENDON STRUCTURE

Tendons consist of densely packed collagen fibrils that are longitudinally oriented. Normal tendons display a fibrillar architecture with ultrasound (Figure 7.1). In general, most tendons have a synovial sheath in areas where they have a curved path across synovial regions near their connection to bone to reduce friction with movement (Figure 7.2). Tendons that have a straight path typically have a paratenon to reduce friction with movement. The paratenon, unlike the tighter synovial sheath, is a loose envelope with adipose and areolar tissue as well as vascular structures. Both structures appear as hyperechoic borders surrounding the tendon but also have different sonographic appearance in both normal and pathologic conditions.

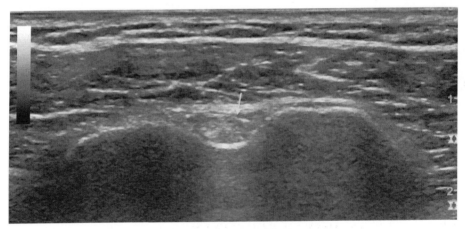

FIGURE 7.1 Sonogram demonstrating a long-axis view of the patellar tendon. The fine fibrillar architecture of the tendon is demonstrated.

(A)

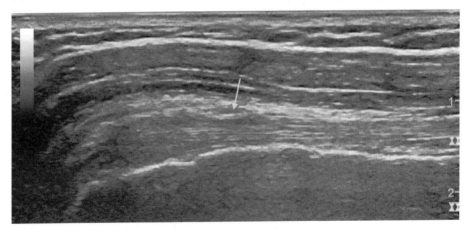

(B)

FIGURE 7.2 Sonograms demonstrating both short-axis (A) and long-axis (B) views of the biceps brachii tendon at the level of its synovial sheath (yellow arrow).

SCANNING TECHNIQUE FOR TENDONS

The tendon should be scanned in both short and long axis (Figure 7.3). The characteristic fibrillar pattern of the tendon should be identified. The appearance of tendons is generally distinct from that seen with the fascicular architecture of peripheral nerves (Figure 7.4).

It is generally helpful to first identify the bony acoustic landmark of the origin or insertion of the tendon for localization (Figure 7.5). This region should be scanned in both long and short axis with the entire footprint of the tendon insertion inspected (Figure 7.6). Most tendons should be viewed from their level of origin or insertion as far as their myotendinous junction (Figure 7.7). Some tendons originate from more than one muscle and each interface should be visualized (Figure 7.8). In addition, some muscles have more than one tendinous origin or insertion, and both areas should be scanned for completeness (Figure 7.9).

The examiner should use purposeful scanning techniques when inspecting tendons. There is a tendency for novice examiners to scan in nonpurposeful swirling motions or other nondirectional patterns. The beam of the transducer is very thin, often roughly the width of a credit card. This creates

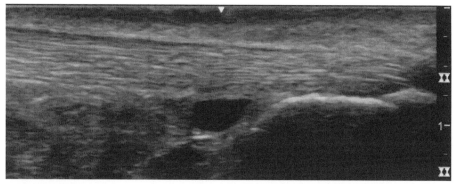

(A)

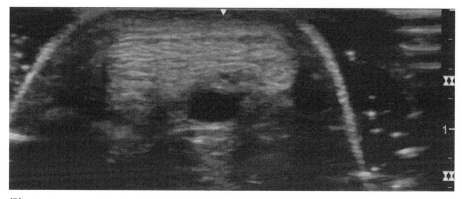

(B)

FIGURE 7.3 Sonograms demonstrating views of an Achilles tendon in both long (A) and short (B) axis.

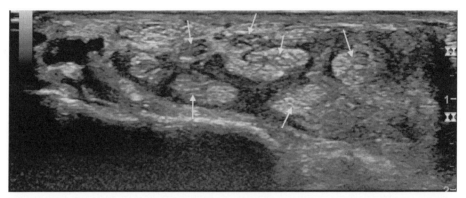

(A)

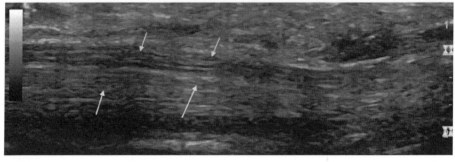

(B)

FIGURE 7.4 Sonograms demonstrating short-axis (A) and long-axis (B) views of the flexor digitorum tendons (yellow arrows) and median nerve (blue arrows) in the carpal tunnel space. The fine fibrillar architecture of the tendons is demonstrated in contrast to the fascicular pattern of the median nerve. Note that in the short-axis view, a bifid median nerve is shown with two sets of nerve fascicles.

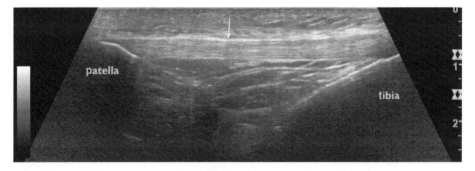

FIGURE 7.5 Sonogram demonstrating a long-axis view of the patellar tendon (yellow arrow). Note the bright bony landmarks of the patella and the tibia.

a longitudinal image of a tendon that displays a considerable amount of length (ie, length of the transducer) but very little width. For this reason, the transducer should be moved back and forth to examine the entire width of the tendon before advancing the transducer to visualize more of the length. The entire width of tendons is seen in short axis, but the scanning motion should be used to assess the length of the tendon.

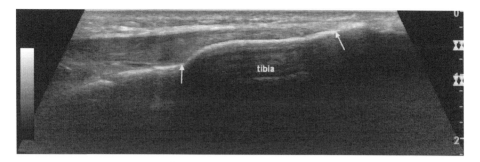

FIGURE 7.6 Sonogram demonstrating a long-axis view of the entire footprint of the insertion of the patellar tendon on the tibia (yellow arrows).

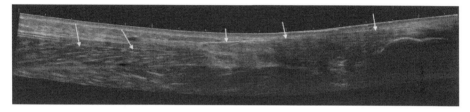

FIGURE 7.7 Extended field of view sonogram demonstrating a long-axis view of the Achilles tendon (yellow arrows) including its insertion on the calcaneus. Also seen is the more proximal myotendinous junction and the soleus (blue arrows).

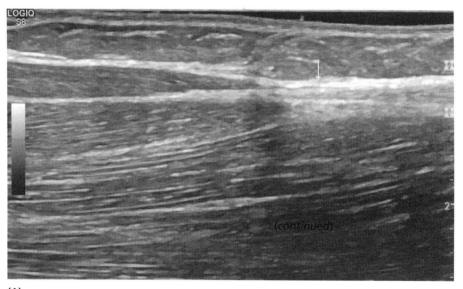

(A)

FIGURE 7.8 Sonograms demonstrating both long-axis (A) and short-axis (B) views of the myotendinous junction of the biceps brachii long head and short head with the common distal tendon. The interface of both muscle tendon junctions should be thoroughly inspected when investigating potential injury.

(continued)

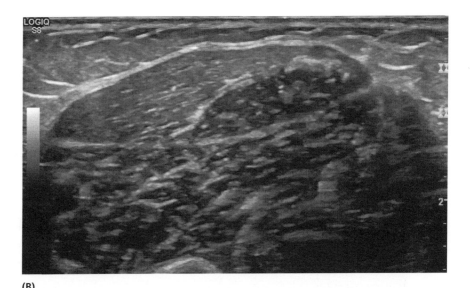

(B)

FIGURE 7.8 *(continued)*

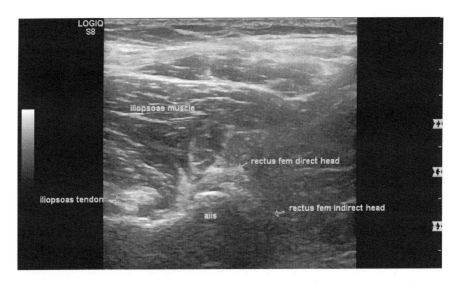

FIGURE 7.9 Sonogram demonstrating a short-axis view of the direct and indirect origins of the rectus femoris from an anterior inferior iliac spine (AIIS). Note that the tendon of the indirect head of the rectus femoris is less conspicuous in this view due to anisotropic artifact because the incident sound beam from the transducer is not orthogonal to its position. The transducer should be moved appropriately to inspect both tendon origins adequately in such circumstances.

Tendons generally have significant anisotropic artifact when the incident sound wave is not orthogonal to the tissue (Figure 4.7). Toggling and heel-to-toe rocking of the transducer should be incorporated into tendon scanning to minimize this artifact. These techniques are discussed in more detail in Chapter 5. To avoid confusion, particularly in beginners, toggling and rocking of the transducer should only be done when the base is stationary (Figure 7.10).

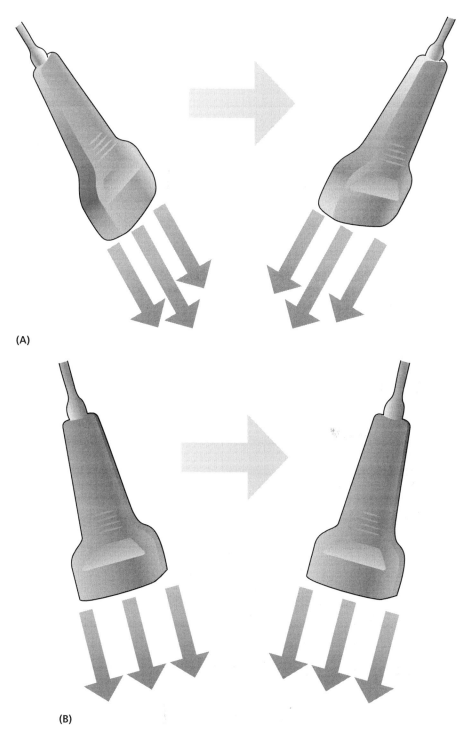

FIGURE 7.10 Illustrations demonstrating toggling (A) and heel-to-toe rocking maneuvers with the transducer (B). These motions are used to alter the direction of the beam from the transducer to create a more perpendicular approach to the tissue desired to reduce anisotropic artifact. These maneuvers are particularly important when inspecting tendons.

TENDON PATHOLOGY

Ultrasound is highly sensitive for detecting diseased or damaged tendon. Tendons can become thickened and more hypoechoic (darker) with degeneration and also display a disruption of the normal architecture. The tendon should be examined for intrasubstance degeneration, enlargement, and tearing (Figure 7.11). Tearing can be partial thickness or full thickness (Figure 7.12). The extent of the tearing should be described in detail and should be examined in both short- and long-axis views. Small foci of hyperechoic signal representing calcification or ossification can be seen in calcific tendonopathy (Figure 7.13).

Tendons should be scanned in their entirety from the bony insertion or origin through its myotendinous junction because injury or degeneration can occur at any point in this complex.

When scanning this region the bony surface should be inspected for irregularity or spurring. This can often represent chronic traction spurring or undersurface tearing. Abnormal tendon thickness and hypoechoic echotecture can reflect enthesopathy at these sites (Figure 7.14). Areas that have a tendon sheath should be inspected for signs of enlargement or fluid, suggesting tenosynovitis (Figure 7.15). Power Doppler can be used to assess for neo-vascularization in chronic tendonopathy. This is often represented by increased flow on Doppler ultrasound (Figure 7.16). Although milder tendon pathology can often be bilateral, it is generally helpful to perform side-to-side comparisons to assess for differences (Figure 7.17).

The interpretation of tendon pathology should always be taken into appropriate clinical context. A focused history and physical for the presenting complaint should be obtained and the relationship of the findings to that information should be considered.

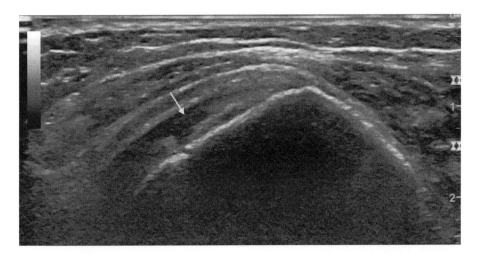

FIGURE 7.11 Sonogram demonstrating a long-axis view of an intrasubstance tear (yellow arrow) in the supraspinatus tendon. The tear is seen as a hypoechoic (dark) area with loss of the normal architecture.

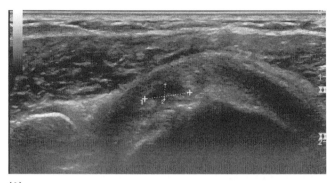

(A)

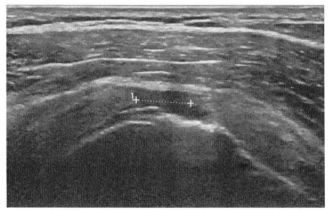

(B)

FIGURE 7.12 Sonograms demonstrating a short-axis view of a partial thickness supraspinatus tear (A) and a long-axis view of a full thickness supraspinatus tear (B).

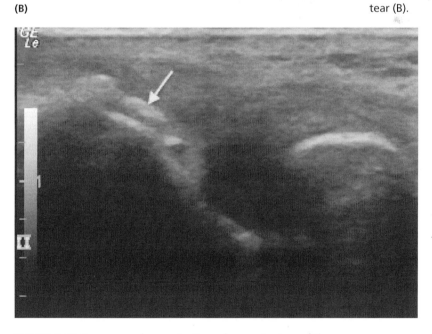

FIGURE 7.13 Sonogram demonstrating a long-axis view of the common extensor tendon with calcific tendonopathy (yellow arrow). The calcifications are seen as the hyperechoic (bright) signal intensity lying outside of the normal bone matrix.

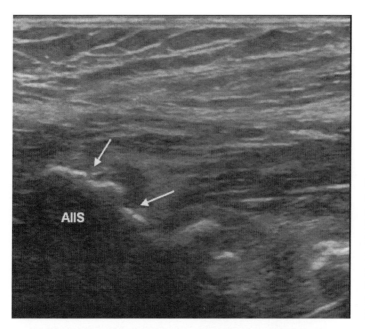

FIGURE 7.14 Sonogram demonstrating enthesopathy of the origin of the direct head of the rectus femoris. Note the irregularity of the bony surfaces of the anterior inferior iliac spine (AIIS) and the abnormal echotecture of the tendon near the bone (yellow arrows).

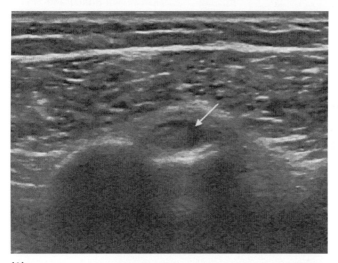

(A)

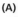

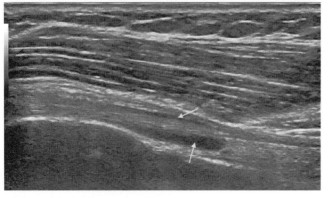

(B)

FIGURE 7.15 Sonograms demonstrating a short-axis (A) and long-axis (B) view of abnormal fluid accumulation (yellow arrows) around the long head of the biceps brachii tendon. The fluid presents as a hypoechoic (dark) or anechoic (black) region around the fibrillar tendon.

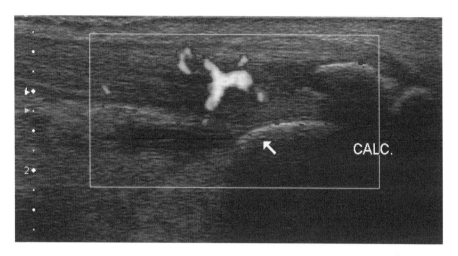

FIGURE 7.16 Sonogram demonstrating a long-axis view of Achilles tendonopathy with increased Doppler flow.

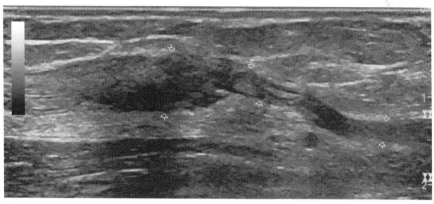

(A)

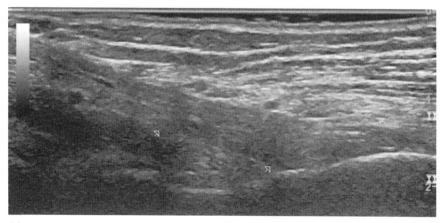

(B)

FIGURE 7.17 Sonograms demonstrating long-axis view of a distal biceps brachii rupture with retraction of tendon fibers (A) and the normal biceps brachii tendon on the contralateral side (B). The side-to-side comparisons demonstrate the dramatic difference between the two tendons.

REMEMBER ·

1) Use the bony acoustic landmarks of the bony origin and insertion to help identify the tendon.
2) Irregularities in the bone or underlying cartilage can often be an indication of tendon injury.
3) Use purposeful movement with the transducer to visualize the entire width of the tendon when in long axis and the appropriate length when in short axis.
4) The transducer beam should be positioned as perpendicular as possible to the tendon to minimize anisotropic artifact.
5) Always consider the appropriate clinical context when interpreting tendon pathology.

BIBLIOGRAPHY

1. Bianchi S, Martinoli C, eds. *Ultrasound of the Musculoskeletal System*. Berlin: Springer-Verlag; 2007.

2. Hartgerink P, Fessell DP, Jacobson JA, van Holsbeeck MT. Full- versus partial thickness Achilles tendon tears: sonographic accuracy and characterization in 26 cases with surgical correlation. *Radiology*. 2001;220:406–412.

3. Jacobson JA. *Fundamentals of Musculoskeletal Ultrasound*. 2nd ed. Philadelphia, PA: Elsevier Saunders; 2013.

4. Smith J, Finnoff JT. Diagnostic and interventional musculoskeletal ultrasound: part 1. Fundamentals. *PM&R*. 2009;1(1):64–75.

5. Van Holsbeeck MT, Introcaso JS. *Musculoskeletal Ultrasound*. 2nd ed. St. Louis, MO: Mosby; 2001.

8

Imaging Muscle

Ultrasound provides high-resolution images of muscle and can detect even subtle abnormalities. The dynamic capabilities of ultrasound allow identification of pathology not appreciable with static imaging. Ultrasound allows precise measurement of muscle size and can detect atrophy as well as echotexture changes in muscle disease.

MUSCLE ARCHITECTURE

Muscles are generally more hypoechoic (darker) relative to other tissues such as tendons (Figure 8.1). Knowledge of muscle anatomy is critical for understanding the region scanned because muscle tissue makes up the majority of the image in the limbs. Muscles have characteristic architecture that includes intervening hypoechoic muscle fibers with hyperechoic connective tissue that creates the perimysium. The short-axis view of muscle has been described as a "starry night" appearance. This image is a result of the hyperechoic (bright) connective tissue interspersed between the hypoechoic (dark) muscle fibers (Figure 8.2). Skeletal muscle is made of individual muscle fibers that are grouped in bundles called a fasciculus (Figure 8.3). Muscle fiber diameter is somewhat smaller than the resolution of current high-frequency ultrasound and ranges from approximately 40 to 80 μm.

There are different types of arrangements of skeletal muscles in the limbs. This includes *pennate, parallel, convergent,* and *quadrilateral*-shaped muscles (Figure 8.4). Pennate muscles that have many fibers per unit area are arranged into three types: unipennate, bipennate, or multipennate (Figure 8.5). Parallel muscles have fibers that run parallel to each other.

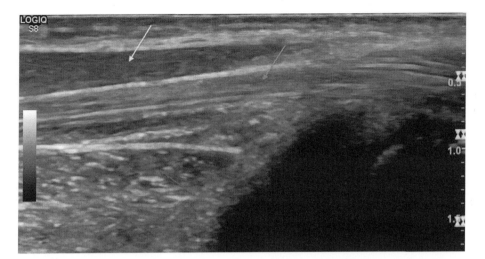

FIGURE 8.1 Sonogram demonstrating the contrast between muscle and tendon. The more hypoechoic (darker) muscle in long axis is demonstrated (yellow arrow) next to the hyperechoic (brighter) tendon in long axis. Note the hypoechoic muscle fibers in relation to the fibrillar architecture of the tendon. Also note the different appearance of muscle oriented in short axis relative to the transducer (red arrow).

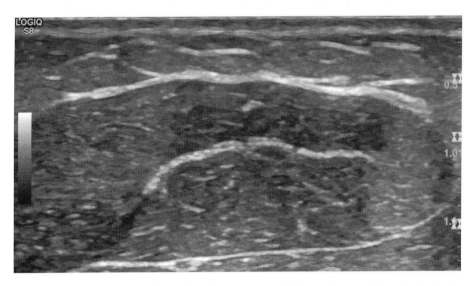

FIGURE 8.2 Sonogram demonstrating the "starry night" appearance of muscle in short axis with intervening bright perimysium interspersed with darker muscle fibers.

When the parallel-shaped muscle bulges in the middle, it is considered *fusiform*. Convergent muscles have fibers that converge at the insertion (Figure 8.6). Quadrilateral-type muscles have fibers in parallel, and are oriented in the same longitudinal axis as the tendon (Figure 8.7). Examples of quadrilateral-type muscles include the pronator quadratus and quadratus plantae. Familiarity with the different arrangement of muscles improves recognition of the muscle landmarks.

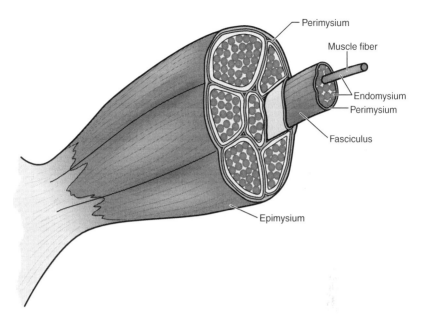

FIGURE 8.3 Illustration of the components of skeletal muscle. The bundle of muscle fibers surrounded by perimysium makes up the fasciculus.

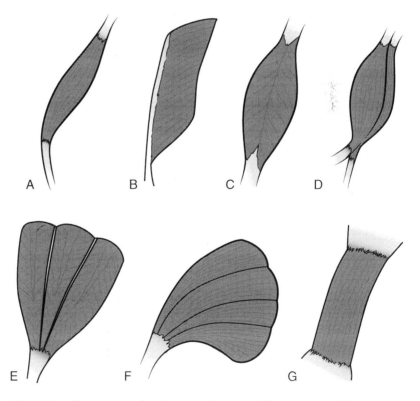

FIGURE 8.4 Illustrations of various muscles types. Shown are parallel (A), unipennate (B), bipennate (C), fusiform (D), multipennate (E), convergent (F), and quadrilateral (G).

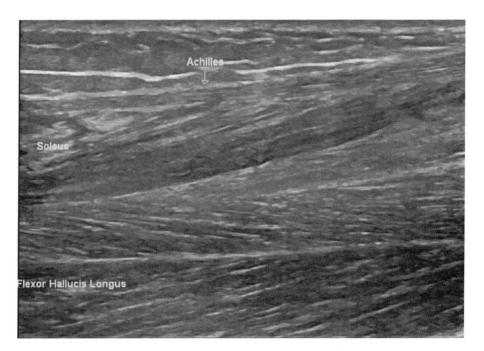

FIGURE 8.5 Sonogram demonstrating the unipennate structure of the soleus inserting on the Achilles tendon. Deep to the bipennate structure of the flexor hallucis longus is shown.

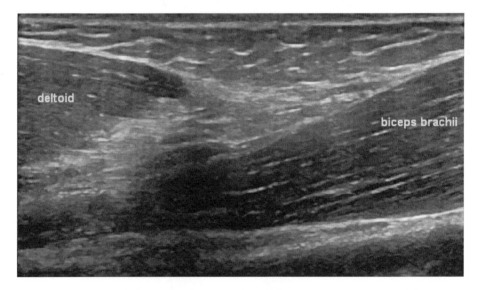

FIGURE 8.6 Sonogram demonstrating a portion of the convergent pattern of the deltoid next to the fusiform pattern of the biceps brachii.

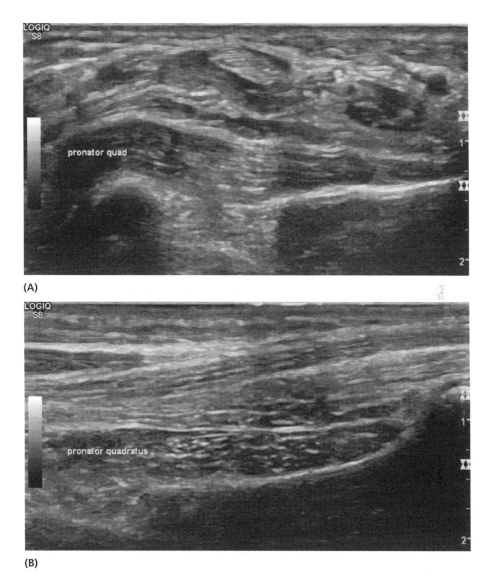

(A)

(B)

FIGURE 8.7 Sonogram demonstrating the quadrilateral-shaped pronator quadratus in long (A) and short (B) axis.

MUSCLE IMAGING TECHNIQUES

Muscle should be scanned in both short and long axis and sufficient area should be inspected to enable pathology to be spotted when present. The transducer should be placed in the proper plane of short and long axis, rather than obliquely to more readily identify the normal architecture (Figure 8.8). Knowledge of the normal shape and location of insertion and origin of the specific muscle being inspected is critical for appropriate transducer placement.

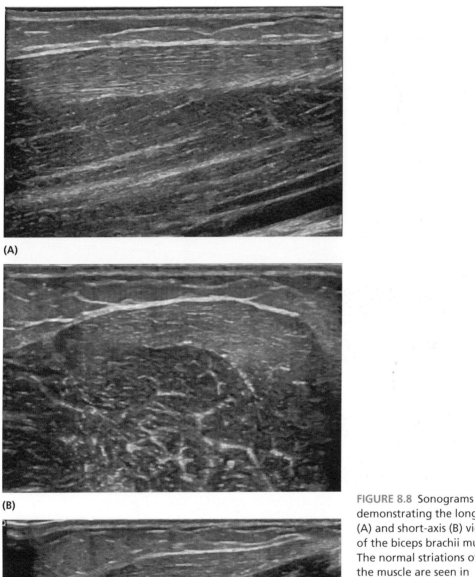

(A)

(B)

(C)

FIGURE 8.8 Sonograms demonstrating the long-axis (A) and short-axis (B) views of the biceps brachii muscle. The normal striations of the muscle are seen in longitudinal view and the cross-sectional architecture is well identified in proper short-axis view. Inspecting the muscle architecture is somewhat more challenging when the transducer is in an oblique position (C) relative to the muscle.

Muscles are generally easier to identify in short-axis view (Figure 8.9). Detailed knowledge of cross-sectional anatomy is necessary for this. Muscles should also generally be followed to the level of their myotendinous junctions, as this is a frequent site of mechanical injury. This is often easier to identify in long axis (Figure 8.10). Use of tendon origins and insertions is also frequently helpful for identification of muscles when needed.

The dynamic capabilities of ultrasound also provide a significant advantage over other imaging modalities for muscle. Muscle movement can be easily seen with ultrasonography. Muscles can be seen to dynamically lengthen with eccentric contraction and shorten and thicken with concentric contraction. This appearance is also dependent upon whether the orientation is in long or short axis.

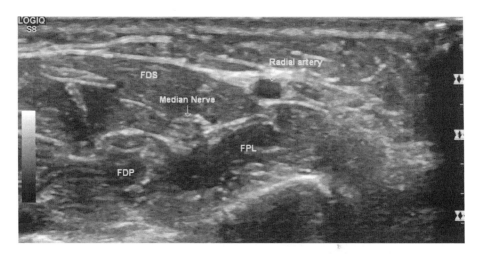

FIGURE 8.9 Sonogram demonstrating a short-axis view of the volar forearm. The short-axis view generally provides the best perspective for locating anatomic landmarks to assist with correctly identifying different muscles. In this view, the flexor digitorum superficialis (FDS), flexor digitorum profundus (FDP), and flexor pollicus longus (FPL) muscles are shown.

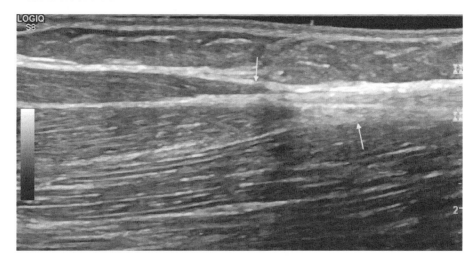

FIGURE 8.10 Sonogram demonstrating a long-axis view of the short and long head of the biceps brachii converging on the more distal tendon. The long-axis view often provides a good perspective when inspecting the myotendinous junction.

MUSCLE PATHOLOGY

Strains

Ultrasound has very good sensitivity for identification of muscle strains. An appropriate history and physical should also be used to assist with localization, however, most muscle strains occur relatively close to the myotendinous junction of the muscle tendon complex (Figure 8.10). Muscles that cross two joints, such as the medial gastrocnemius, rectus femoris, and biceps femoris, are particularly susceptible to injury. Higher grade strains that involve fascia as well as the muscle fibers are easier to identify (Figure 8.11). Lower grade

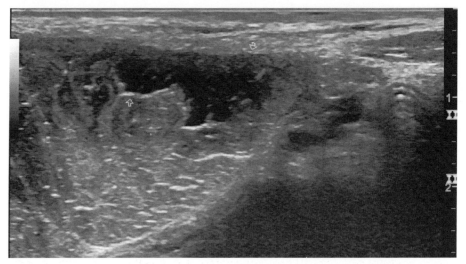

(A)

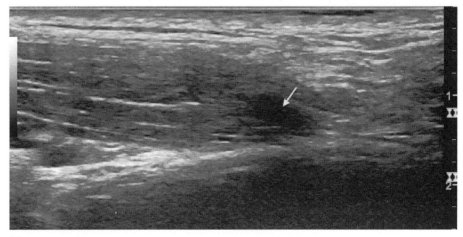

(B)

FIGURE 8.11 Sonograms demonstrating a relatively acute and high grade strain of the rectus abdominus in both short-axis view (A) and long-axis view (B). The muscle defect is seen by the hypoechoic (dark) and irregular signal (yellow arrows) where there is loss of the normal muscle echotexture.

strains that involve only a few muscle fibers require meticulous technique and survey in conjunction with the clinical assessment (Figure 8.12). Muscle strains in general are identified by a disruption of the muscle fibers and normal fibroadipose septa. In acute strains, the injured area typically becomes more hypoechoic (darker) as a result of the infiltration of blood and edema. Confirmation of the abnormality should always be performed in two views (Figure 8.13). Development of the hypoechoic blood and edema infiltration generally takes one to two days after the injury. For this reason, scanning an acute injury too early after onset can have less sensitivity in lower grade injuries. Large hematomas associated with muscle injuries are typically easier to identify and often persist for many weeks (Figure 8.14). More chronic muscle strains can develop fibrotic scarring that manifests as hyperechoic (bright) irregular pattern within the muscle (Figure 8.15).

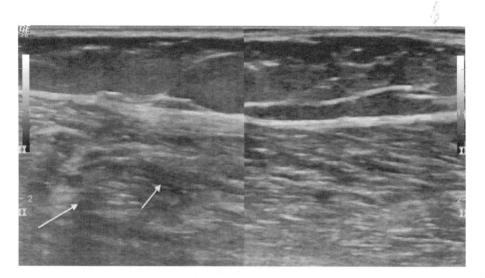

FIGURE 8.12 Sonogram demonstrating an acute relatively low-grade muscle strain (image on the left) in contrast to the unaffected side (image on the right). There is mild disruption of the muscle fibers and normal fibroadipose septa seen with the image on the left (yellow arrows). The change in muscle fiber echotexture is more conspicuous with live dynamic scanning and somewhat harder to detect with still images.

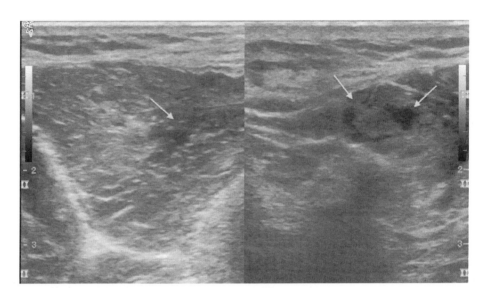

FIGURE 8.13 Sonogram demonstrating an acute latissimus dorsi muscle strain injury in short axis (image on the left) and long axis (image on the right). The strain injury is represented by the hypoechoic (dark) signal and loss of echotexture (yellow arrows). Both short- and long-axis views should always be obtained when assessing tissue injuries of this nature. Frequently one view can be more revealing than the other.

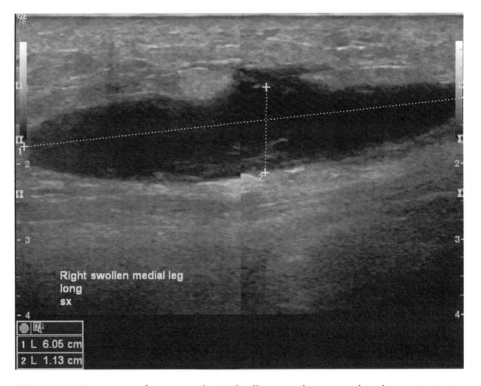

FIGURE 8.14 Sonogram of an approximated split-screen image used to demonstrate a large calf hematoma.

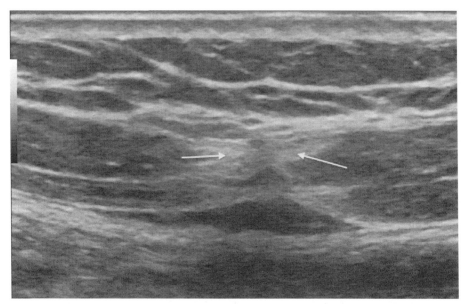

(A)

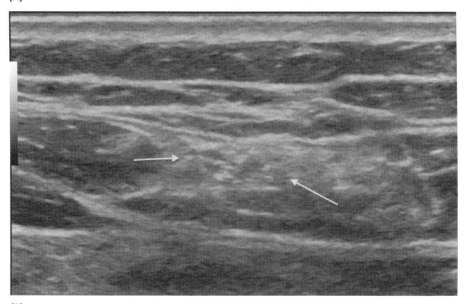

(B)

FIGURE 8.15 Sonograms demonstrating chronic scar (yellow arrows) in both long-axis view (A) and short-axis view (B) from a rectus abdominus strain. The scarring appears as irregular hyperechoic (bright) signal that is in stark contrast to the regular echotexture of the more hypoechoic (dark) muscle tissue.

Postsurgical or Traumatic Alteration

External trauma can occur to muscle in multiple ways. This can be from direct contusion or partial or complete muscle laceration. Hematoma can be present after an external injury and is often identified by hypoechoic (dark) or anechoic (black) appearance (Figure 8.14). In laceration injuries, including surgical changes, the injury pattern can typically be followed from the superior portion of the image through the more superficial tissue (Figure 8.16). Detailed history and physical can help tremendously when assessing the implication of the imaging findings in the setting of prior surgery or trauma.

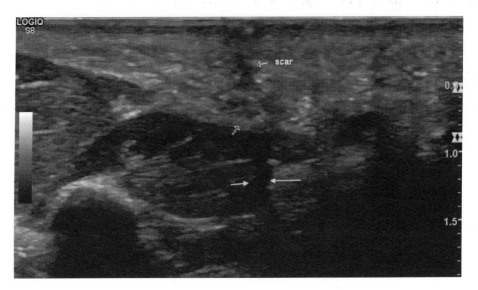

FIGURE 8.16 Sonogram demonstrating the irregular disruption of the muscle fibers (blue arrows). The more superficial tissue scar is also shown (yellow arrows).

Muscle Hernias

Muscle hernias are a focal defect in the muscle fascia that results in a protrusion of muscle through the defect. They can be asymptomatic but also a source of pain. Some seek evaluation for the concerns of a possible mass. Ultrasound is the imaging modality of choice for muscle hernias (Figure 8.17). The examiner should use plenty of conduction gel and only light pressure with the transducer. Hernias are usually more evident when the muscle is under contraction.

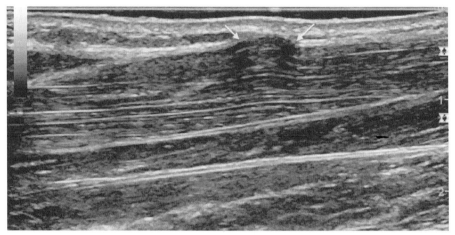

(A)

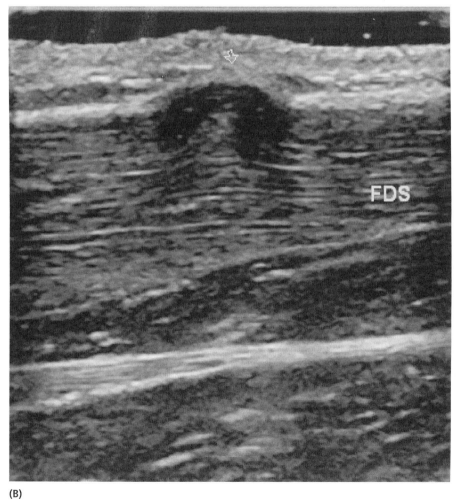

(B)

FIGURE 8.17 Sonograms showing a long-axis view of a muscle herniation (yellow arrows). The image in (A) shows the muscle under slight contraction and the image in (B) shows the muscle under a more vigorous contraction.

Denervation

Injury to muscle innervation leads to denervation atrophy. This is seen on ultrasound in more chronic conditions as more hyperechoic (brighter) echotexture as a result of muscle tissue gradually being replaced by fatty tissue (Figure 8.18). It is also an effect of an increased ratio of connective tissue relative to viable muscle fibers. In addition, neurogenic atrophy results in loss of size of the involved muscle (Figure 8.19). Side-to-side comparisons

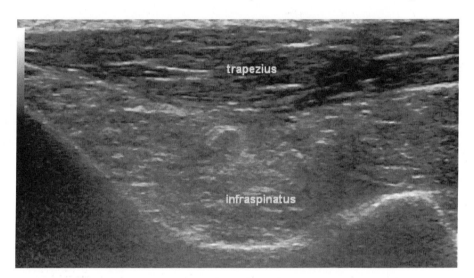

FIGURE 8.18 Sonogram demonstrating the hyperechoic (bright) appearance of an infraspinatus in short axis with denervation from a suprascapular neuropathy. Note the contrast of the normal echotexture of trapezius.

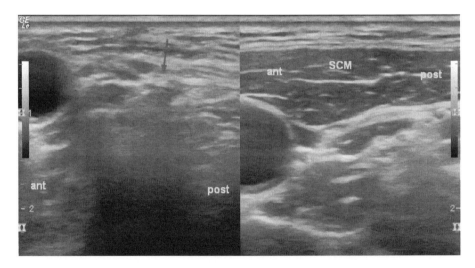

FIGURE 8.19 Sonogram demonstrating a short-axis view of a sternocleidomastoid (SCM) with denervation atrophy (image on the left, red arrow) in contrast to the unaffected side (image on the right). Note that the muscle with denervation has lost its normal muscle echotexture and this has been replaced by hyperechoic (bright) connective tissue.

of muscle are often very helpful to assess unilateral peripheral motor nerve injuries (Figure 8.20). The comparisons can provide good perspective on the echotexture changes and precise measurements can be made for comparing the size.

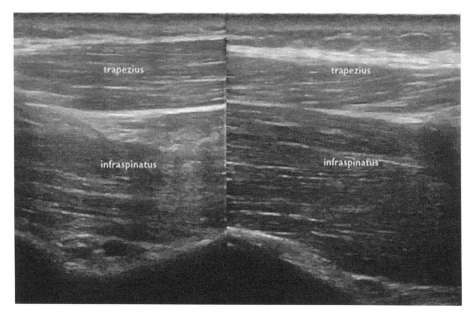

FIGURE 8.20 Sonogram demonstrating a short-axis view of an infraspinatus muscle with partial denervation (image on the left) in contrast with the normal side on the right. In this case, the neuropathy is not severe to the extent that there is complete loss of muscle substance. The use of side-to-side comparisons allows the identification of a more hyperechoic (brighter) appearance of the muscle on the affected side.

Myopathy

Muscle abnormalities are different in most myopathies than in neurogenic denervation. Similar to neurogenic atrophy, the muscle echotexture is generally more hyperechoic (bright) compared to normal muscle (Figure 8.21). This is due to the loss of normal muscle tissue as well as the interposition of fatty tissue, fibrosis and in some circumstances, inflammatory mediators. A difference from neurogenic atrophy is that in myopathy, there is usually relative preservation of muscle size. Most myopathies are generalized and relatively symmetrical so side-to-side comparisons are rarely helpful and the muscle echotexture should generally be compared to an established standard reference when available. Some myopathies have focal areas of relative involvement and sparing, which can be readily distinguished on ultrasound. This makes ultrasound a useful tool for determining areas of involvement, which can help with myopathy identification.

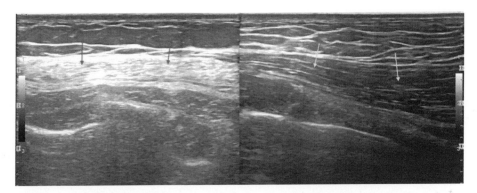

FIGURE 8.21 Split-screen image sonogram demonstrating the difference in muscle echotexture in an individual with fascio-scapular humeral dystrophy (FSH) (image on the left) compared to that seen in an unaffected individual (image on the right). Note the hyperechoic (bright) appearance of the muscle of the individual with FSH (red arrows) relative to the normal comparison (yellow arrows).

Anomolous, Congenitally Absent, and Accessory Muscles

Anomolous, accessory, or congenitally absent muscles are not considered pathologic; however, their identification can provide clarification in pathologic circumstances. Patients are often unaware of these variations unless there is abnormal shape causing concern for tumor. Muscles are considered anomalous when they are in a pattern that is a variant of normal anatomy. They are considered accessory when they are additional muscles that are not normally present (Figure 8.22). Ultrasound can be helpful in distinguishing congenitally absent muscles from atrophy and denervation. In all of these circumstances, a detailed knowledge of muscle anatomy, including the normal origins and insertions, and common anatomic variation, is needed in

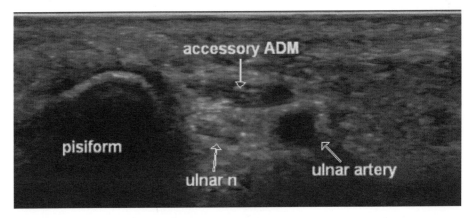

FIGURE 8.22 Sonogram demonstrating an example of an accessory muscle that can be identified with ultrasound. The image is a short-axis view of the ulnar tunnel with an accessory abductor digiti minimi muscle (accessory ADM) seen as a hypoechoic area of muscle overlying the neurovascular structures.

combination with good scanning technique to make accurate conclusions. As with other tissue inspected in a musculoskeletal evaluation, any pathologic findings should always be considered with an appropriate clinical context with information gained in the history and physical examination.

REMEMBER

1) Muscles are generally more hypoechoic (darker) than other tissue.
2) Scanning muscle to the level of its origin and insertion can assist in identification.
3) Muscle pathology should always be assessed in both short- and long-axis planes.
4) Muscle pathology should always be interpreted within appropriate clinical context.

BIBLIOGRAPHY

1. Bianchi S, Martinoli C, eds. *Ultrasound of the Musculoskeletal System*. Berlin: Springer-Verlag; 2007.

2. Jacobson JA. *Fundamentals of Musculoskeletal Ultrasound*. 2nd ed. Philadelphia, PA: Elsevier Saunders; 2013.

3. Strakowski JA. *Ultrasound Evaluation of Focal Neuropathies. Correlation With Electrodiagnosis*. New York, NY: Demos Medical; 2014.

4. Van Holsbeeck MT, Introcaso JS. *Musculoskeletal Ultrasound*. 2nd ed. St. Louis, MO: Mosby; 2001.

5. Walker FO, Cartwright MS, Wiesler ER, Caress J. Ultrasound of nerve and muscle. *Clin Neurophysiol*. 2004;115(3):495–507.

CHAPTER 9

Imaging Nerve

Ultrasound is an excellent modality for evaluation of peripheral nerve tissue. The high resolution and dynamic capabilities allow precise measurements of even subtle changes, detection of alteration of the internal structure, and dynamic effect of surrounding tissue. Developing skills for imaging peripheral nerves can be used for proper tissue recognition in musculoskeletal evaluations, diagnostic assessment of both focal and generalized neuropathies, and in identification for nerve blocks.

NORMAL NERVE ARCHITECTURE

The appearance of nerve on ultrasound is that of an uninterrupted fascicular pattern (Figure 9.1). This differs from the intercalated pattern typical of tendons (Figure 9.2). The hypoechoic (dark) nerve fascicles are seen among the hyperechoic (bright) epineurium. In short-axis view, this creates an appearance that is frequently described as resembling a "honeycomb" (Figure 9.3).

Histologically, the fascicles are enveloped by perineurium and the nerve fibers are covered by endoneurium (Figure 9.4). The outer sheath is termed the epineurium or "outer epineurium" and the tissue between the fascicles and the outer epineurium is sometimes referred to as the "inner epineurium."

Nerves often have arteries and veins that accompany them and it is necessary to recognize them for reliable identification (Figure 9.5). Doppler imaging can be used to attempt to see flow in suspected vessels (Figure 9.6). Veins can be identified by their compressibility (Figure 9.7). Nerves generally have intraneural vessels; however, these are usually not readily identifiable on

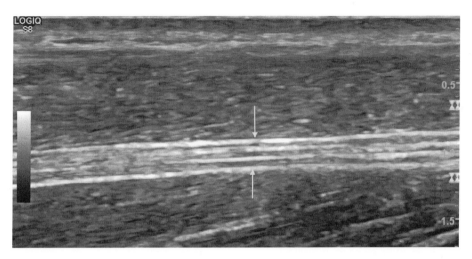

FIGURE 9.1 Sonogram demonstrating a long-axis view of the uninterrupted fascicular pattern of normal nerve (yellow arrows).

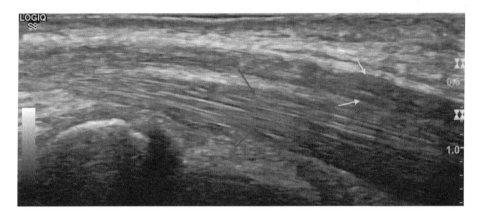

FIGURE 9.2 Sonogram demonstrating a long-axis view of the fine intercalated fibrillar pattern of a tendon (red arrows) in contrast to the fascicular pattern of a nerve (yellow arrows).

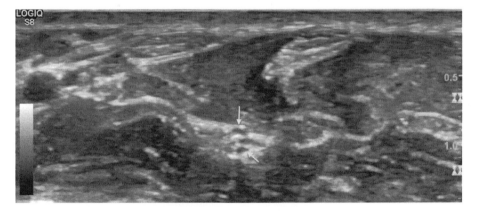

FIGURE 9.3 Sonogram demonstrating a nerve (yellow arrows) in short-axis view. Note the hypoechoic (dark) round fascicles surrounded by the hyperechoic epineurium.

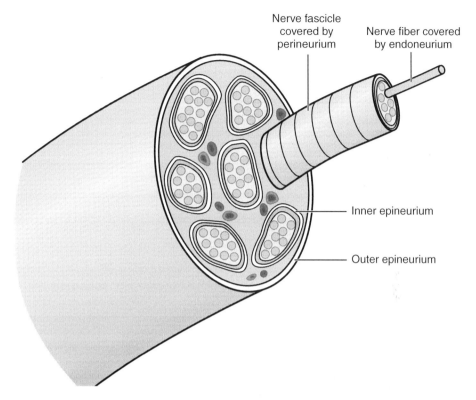

FIGURE 9.4 Illustration of the components of a peripheral nerve, demonstrating the nerve fiber covered by the endoneurium, the nerve fascicle covered by the perineurium, and the groups of fascicles covered by the epineurium.

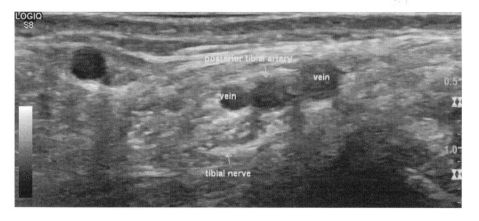

FIGURE 9.5 Sonogram demonstrating a short-axis view of the tibial nerve at the level of the ankle. The accompanying posterior tibial artery and veins can be used to help identify the nerve.

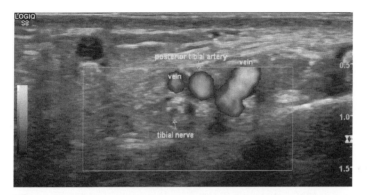

(A)

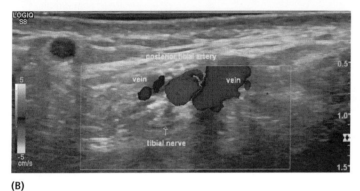

(B)

FIGURE 9.6 Sonograms demonstrating the use of power (A) and color (B) Doppler to identify the tibial artery and veins. Flow is created through the veins by changing the amount of pressure from the transducer.

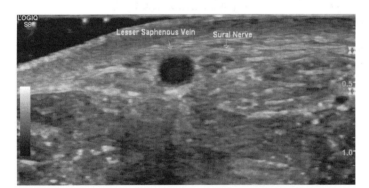

(A)

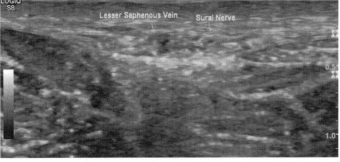

(B)

FIGURE 9.7 Sonograms demonstrating a short-axis view of the sural nerve. The hypoechoic (dark) lesser saphenous vein is used as a landmark to identify the nerve. Note that the vein is highly visible with less transducer pressure (A) but is compressed and less conspicuous with more transducer pressure (B).

ultrasound. It is important to reliably identify the larger vascular structures so that they are distinguished from the nerve when performing measurements. Often, scanning proximally and distally can improve this determination. Use of Doppler is also helpful when needed (Figure 9.8).

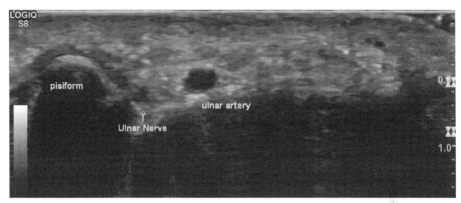

(A)

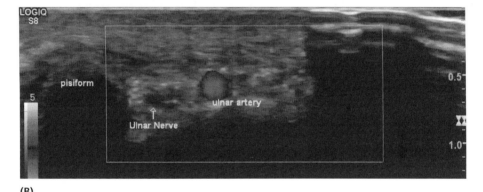

(B)

FIGURE 9.8 Sonograms of a short-axis view of the ulnar nerve at the ulnar tunnel. The gray scale image (A) shows the nerve and artery both appear hypoechoic (dark) relative to the surrounding tissue. The use of Doppler (B) helps distinguish the ulnar artery from the nerve.

NERVE SCANNING TECHNIQUES

Nerves are generally easier to identify in short-axis view. Efforts should be made to identify the fascicular architecture and distinguish it from the surrounding tissue (Figure 9.9). Scanning back and forth can help distinguish the nerve tissue from other surrounding tissue. Other techniques used to improve the conspicuity of the nerve include movement of the surrounding tissue, rocking or toggling the transducer, or moving to a position where there is more contrast from the surrounding tissue relative to the nerve (Figure 9.10). Using conspicuous anatomic landmarks can help identify the location of more challenging nerves (Figure 9.11). When following the

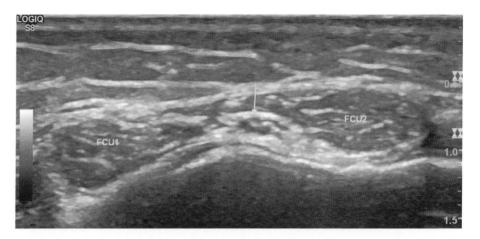

FIGURE 9.9 Sonogram demonstrating a short-axis view of the ulnar nerve in the cubital tunnel. The nerve tissue is distinguished from the surrounding muscle tissue, in this case the two heads of the flexor carpi ulnaris (FCU1, FCU2). Following the nerve back and forth in short axis can help increase conspicuity by accentuating the contrast relative to other tissue.

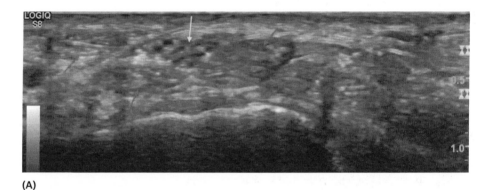

(A)

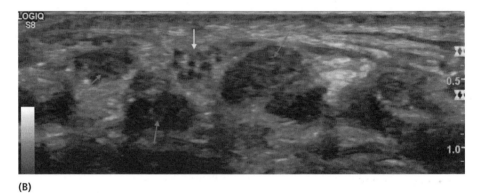

(B)

FIGURE 9.10 Sonograms demonstrating the use of anisotropy to help distinguish nerve tissue from tendon. The images demonstrate a short-axis view of the median nerve (yellow arrows) and surrounding flexor tendons (red arrows) in the carpal tunnel. Image (A) demonstrates the appearance with the transducer orthogonal to the nerve and tendons. In image (B), the transducer is toggled, decreasing the anisotropic artifact of the tissue. Note that the anisotropic artifact is considerably greater with the tendons resulting in a more dramatic change in echotexture. This illustrates how toggling the transducer can increase the conspicuity of the nerve.

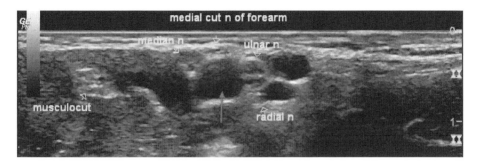

FIGURE 9.11 Sonogram demonstrating an example of identifying more challenging nerves based on another anatomic landmark. The different peripheral nerves are identified based on their position in relation to the axillary artery (red arrow).

course of a nerve in short axis, it is often more effective to scan rapidly rather than too slowly to accentuate the contrast in tissue. Using liberal amounts of coupling gel is helpful to facilitate that.

The examiner should be vigilant about the amount of pressure that is being placed on the tissue by the transducer. Excessive pressure can alter the shape of the underlying nerve as well as compress the surrounding tissue. This includes surrounding vascular structures such as veins that can often help with localization (Figure 9.7). In some circumstances, the use of higher transducer pressure can improve the image quality of a relatively deep nerve (Figure 9.12).

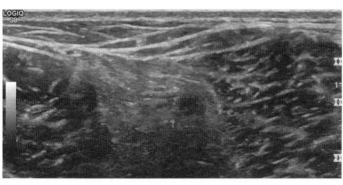

(A)

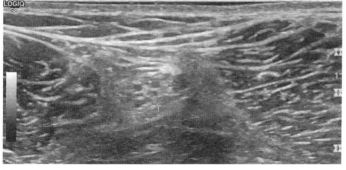

(B)

FIGURE 9.12 Sonograms of short-axis views of the same sciatic nerve (yellow arrows) demonstrating the potential benefit of increased transducer pressure. The image in (A) is with light transducer pressure and the image in (B) has increased transducer pressure. Note the increased resolution of the fascicular architecture of the deep sciatic nerve with the increased transducer pressure (B).

Nerves can also be precisely measured with most ultrasound instruments. Cross-sectional area measurements of nerves in short axis are the most commonly used. This can be performed both by direct tracing inside the border of the nerve or more indirectly by the use of calipers and an ellipse. With either technique, the measurement should be performed on the inner aspect of the outer epineurium (Figure 9.13). Once adequate experience has been gained, the direct tracing method is generally preferable for reliability. Care should be used to establish that the measurement of the nerve is being obtained with the image as perpendicular as possible to obtain a reliable measurement. This usually means that the transducer should be oriented to create the smallest cross-sectional area possible while maintaining a short-axis plain. Obliquity of the image can create an artifactually inaccurate large cross-sectional area (Figure 9.14). With nerves that are relatively small in size,

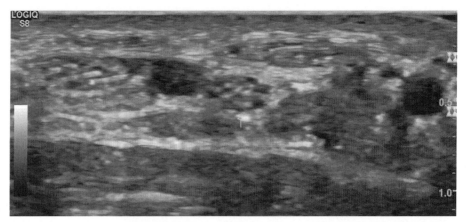

(A)

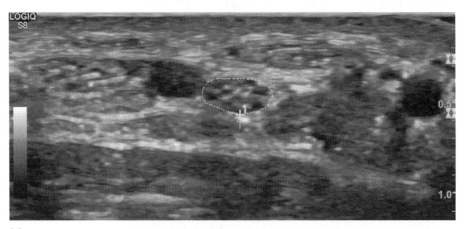

(B)

FIGURE 9.13 Sonograms of short-axis views of a nerve. The image in (A) is the nerve with the transducer place in perpendicular position noted by the smallest cross-sectional area. The image in (B) is the same picture with the nerve measured using the direct tracing method. Note that the trace is at the inner border of the outer epineurium.

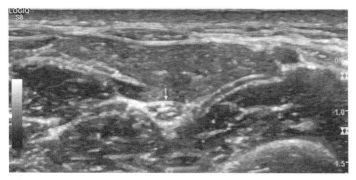

(A)

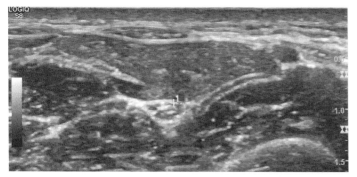

(B)

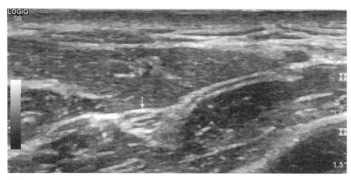

(C)

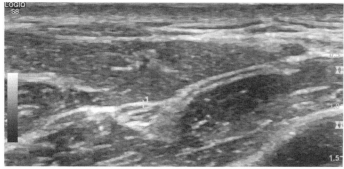

(D)

FIGURE 9.14 Sonograms of short-axis views of the median nerve in the forearm. The image in (A) demonstrates the nerve with the transducer in the proper perpendicular position and (B) shows the direct tracing for cross-sectional area of that image. The image in (C) demonstrates the nerve with the transducer in a somewhat oblique position to the nerve creating an appearance of an abnormally large cross-sectional area. The image in (D) shows the direct tracing method with the oblique image. These images illustrate the importance of being precisely perpendicular to the nerve to obtain accurate cross-sectional area measurements.

measurement of the diameter in short axis rather than cross-sectional area is more practical because reliable cross-sectional area cannot be obtained.

The diameter is also used for measurement of nerves in long-axis view (Figure 9.15). Measurement in this plane is often more challenging because the nerves often do not follow a straight course. The nerve should be scanned sufficiently to establish that the transducer is appropriately aligned over the maximum diameter of the nerve. The surrounding region should be assessed to reliably confirm that only nerve tissue is being measured. The diameter measurements should also be correlated with those obtained in short-axis view to confirm accuracy.

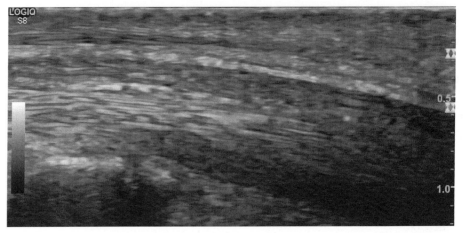

(A)

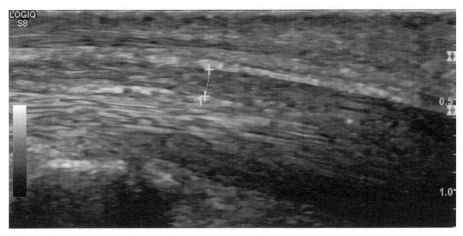

(B)

FIGURE 9.15 Sonograms of a long-axis view of the median nerve (A) as well as a view of the same image with diameter measurement (B).

NERVE PATHOLOGY

The appearance of peripheral nerves on ultrasound due to focal injury or generalized disease can be variable and is often related to the extent of the pathology. Focal neuropathies often present with abnormal swelling that is usually just proximal to the site of the injury (Figure 9.16). However, there can be some variation in the presentation (Figure 9.17). Precise measurements and use of side-to-side comparisons when appropriate can be helpful. The measurements most frequently used are in short axis but long-axis views also provide needed perspective. At the current time, there is considerable variation between published normal values with respect to cross-sectional areas with many peripheral nerves. This seems to reflect variation in the manner in which the nerves are measured, among other factors. The median nerve at the carpal tunnel has been the most frequently studied nerve with ultrasound. Many studies of the median nerve have established slightly different normal values, but there is general consensus that a cross-sectional area of greater than 13 mm^2 is highly predictive for the presence of median neuropathy at the carpal tunnel. Many feel that a cross-sectional area in the realm of 10 to 13 mm^2 is also abnormal. Ultrasound also has sensitivity for identifying median neuropathy that is relatively similar to electrodiagnostic studies. Ultrasound, to this point, has not been shown to be as valuable as electrodiagnosis for determining the relative severity of neuropathies.

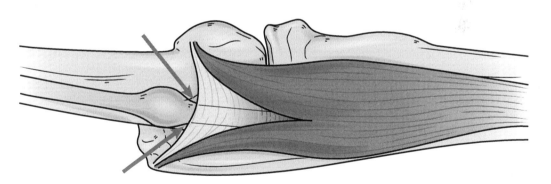

FIGURE 9.16 Illustration of a nerve entrapment. The nerve shows focal enlargement just proximal to the entrapment site (red arrows).

Peripheral nerve size has variation with body mass index, gender, age, and other factors. Using unaffected areas of a peripheral nerve for reference can be helpful in determining pathology (Figure 9.18).

In addition to size measurement, identification of changes in the normal architecture of the nerve can also reveal neuropathy (Figure 9.19). There is

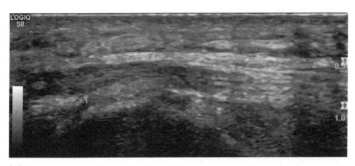

(A)

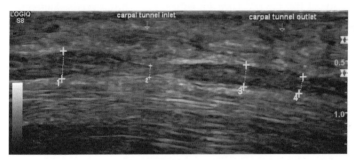

(B)

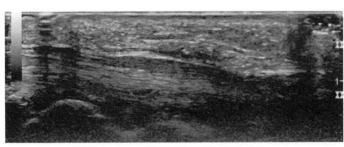

(C)

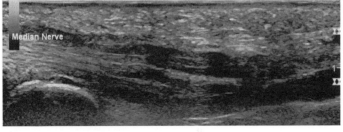

(D)

FIGURE 9.17 Sonograms demonstrating long-axis views of nerve swelling in different entrapment neuropathies. The image in (A) shows a typical entrapment pattern with an ulnar neuropathy at the elbow with distal constriction (superior yellow arrow to the right) and a more proximal focal enlargement (inferior yellow arrow to the left). The other images show postoperative median neuropathy at the carpal tunnel. In (B), there is focal constriction from scarring in the middle and enlargement both proximally and distally to that level. The image in (C) shows a diffuse enlargement in between two areas of focal constriction. In (D), the median nerve is diffusely swollen with multiple areas of tethering from scar. These images demonstrate examples of different presentations of focal neuropathies and reflect the need to examine the entire area of potential pathology.

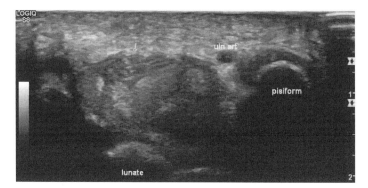

(A)

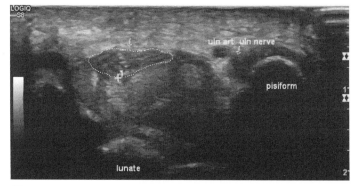

(B)

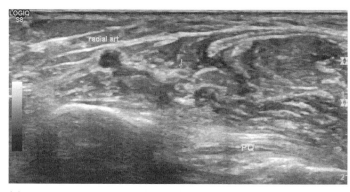

(C)

FIGURE 9.18 Sonograms demonstrating short-axis views of the median nerve (yellow arrow) in an individual with median nerve at the carpal tunnel. The image in (A) shows the median nerve at the carpal tunnel and (B) shows the direct tracing method for calculating the cross-sectional area. The image in (C) shows the median nerve at the level of the distal forearm in the region of the pronator quadratus (PQ). The image in (D) shows the direct tracing of the nerve at this level. The use of an unaffected area, in this case the distal forearm, helps illustrate the relative degree of abnormality seen at the site of entrapment.

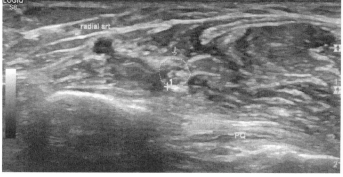

(D)

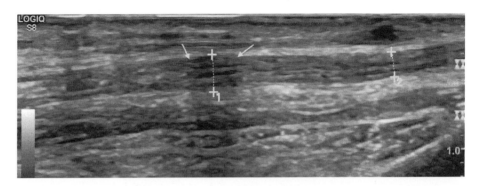

FIGURE 9.19 Sonogram demonstrating a long-axis view of a focal median neuropathy (yellow arrows) in the distal forearm from a crush injury. Note that there is relatively minimal swelling at the area of injury but significant enlargement of the fascicular architecture.

no consistently good correlation between the size of nerves and relative severity of the neuropathy, but visual disruption of the normal fascicular architecture is more often associated with axonal injury. Complete transection of the nerve (neurotmesis) can typically be distinguished from a nonfunctional nerve with the connective tissue intact (complete axonotmesis) on ultrasound (Figure 9.20). This is an advantage of ultrasound over routine physical examination and electrophysiologic studies, which cannot reliably distinguish these conditions. This determination can enhance acumen for treatment decisions, including surgical intervention.

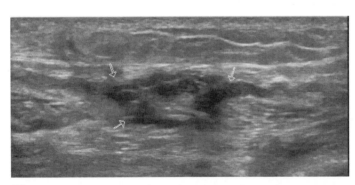

(A)

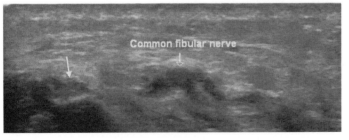

(B)

FIGURE 9.20 Sonograms demonstrating long-axis views of injuries to peripheral nerves. Ultrasound can often demonstrate the difference between a functional axonotmesis with connective tissue still in continuity (A) and a complete neurotmesis where the connective tissue is not in continuity (B). Note in (B) that the nerve tissue is separated (yellow arrows). This is an important feature of imaging tools such as ultrasound, because this distinction cannot be reliably made with conventional electrodiagnostic techniques.

Ultrasound can also identify factors that can be the source of peripheral nerve injuries. This includes intrinsic and extrinsic tumors, abnormal movement and subluxations, encroaching tissue, hematoma, scar and other postsurgical changes, as well as foreign bodies. In addition increased vascularity can be seen in some peripheral nerve lesions with Doppler imaging. Ultrasound is a valuable tool for assessment of peripheral nerves in a vast array of predisposing conditions. As with other tissues inspected in a musculoskeletal or neuromuscular evaluation, pathologic findings should always be considered within the appropriate clinical context, including the information derived from the history and physical examination.

REMEMBER

1) Peripheral nerves have a fascicular architecture that differs from the fibrillar architecture of tendons.
2) Use easy to recognize anatomic landmarks when attempting to visualize nerves that are challenging to identify.
3) Short-axis measurements of peripheral nerves should be made at the inner border of the outer epineurium.
4) Peripheral nerves should always be measured in both short and long axis when distinguishing pathology.
5) Assessment of peripheral nerve pathology should always be considered in the appropriate clinical context.

BIBLIOGRAPHY

1. Bacigalupo L, Bianchi S, Valle M, Martinoli C. [Ultrasonography of peripheral nerves]. *Radiologe*. 2003;43(10):841–849.

2. Bianchi S, Martinoli C, eds. *Ultrasound of the Musculoskeletal System*. Berlin: Springer-Verlag; 2007.

3. Strakowski JA. *Ultrasound Evaluation of Focal Neuropathies. Correlation With Electrodiagnosis*. New York, NY: Demos Medical; 2014.

4. Walker FO, Cartwright MS, Wiesler ER, Caress J. Ultrasound of nerve and muscle. *Clin Neurophysiol*. 2004;115(3):495–507.

CHAPTER 10

Imaging of Other Tissues

INTRODUCTION

Knowledge of the sonographic appearance of other tissues is needed to appropriately identify structural relationships. Bone, skin, fat, cartilage, ligaments, arteries, and veins all have characteristic appearance on ultrasound. Learning the typical and pathologic appearance of these tissues is essential for improving diagnostic acumen with the musculoskeletal ultrasound evaluation.

BONE

Ultrasound waves do not penetrate bone. Because of the densely calcified cortex, virtually all of the sound waves reflect back to the transducer. This high acoustic impedance of bone in relation to surrounding tissue results in a very bright appearance on ultrasound (Figure 10.1). Despite the relatively easy identification of bone with ultrasound, essentially only the cortex surface is reliably visualized. The appearance of the image beneath the cortex of the bone is often referred to as *bone shadow*. This term is used for the acoustic artifact deep to the hyperechoic bone outline that is the result of the sound wave attenuation. This is a limitation of ultrasound because bone tissue and other tissue deep to bone are not adequately visualized. Other imaging modalities such as plain radiographs, computerized tomography, or magnetic resonance imaging should be considered when detailed visualization of bone or soft tissue deep to bone is needed.

Because of their high degree of conspicuity, bony landmarks often provide assistance in identifying soft tissue structures that are more difficult to visualize (Figure 10.2). Abnormalities on the surface of bone, particularly at the interface of ligaments or tendons, often provide clues for injury (Figure 10.3). Ultrasound is an excellent modality for identifying osteophytes and spurs (Figure 10.4) and also has a high resolution for identifying disruptions in the bone cortex that might not be visible on x-ray (Figure 10.5).

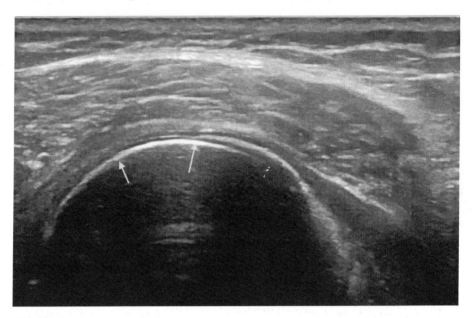

FIGURE 10.1 Sonogram demonstrating the interface of bone (yellow arrows). The difference in impedance between the bone cortex and the surrounding soft tissue results in the hyperechoic appearance.

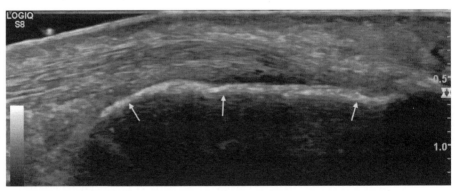

(A)

FIGURE 10.2 Sonograms demonstrating examples of bony landmarks that assist in localization. In (A), the cortex of the calcaneus (yellow arrows) is seen at the insertion of the Achilles tendon in long axis. In (B), a bony landmark on the dorsum of the wrist known as Lister's tubercle (yellow arrows) assists in identifying the dorsal compartments (blue arrows).

(continued)

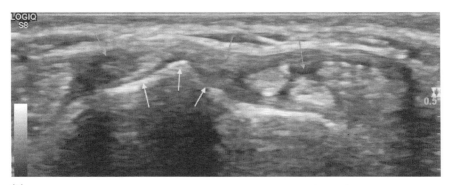

(B)

FIGURE 10.2 (*continued*)

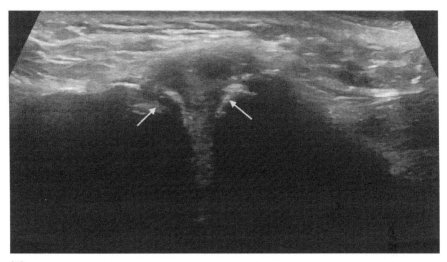

(A)

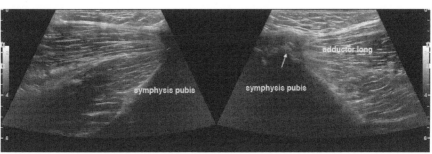

(B)

FIGURE 10.3 Sonograms demonstrating examples of bony irregularity that provide clues for pathology. In (A), the irregular edges of the acromial–clavicular joint are shown (yellow arrows) reflecting a degree of degenerative joint disease. The images in (B) show the irregular edge of the bony origin of the adductor longus demonstrated in long axis (image on the right: yellow arrow), reflecting enthesopathy, in contrast to the relatively normal comparison side (image on the left). The image in (C) shows mild bony irregularity under the insertion of the infraspinatus (yellow arrow). Bony changes of that nature should alert the examiner to inspect for tendonopathy and partial thickness tears in that region.

(continued)

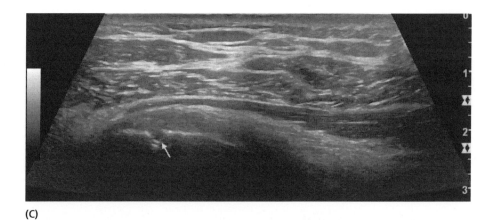

(C)

FIGURE 10.3 (*continued*)

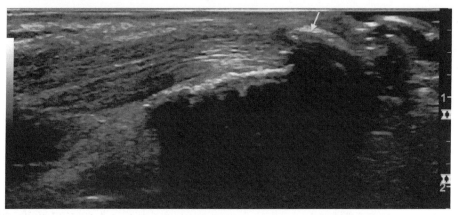

(A)

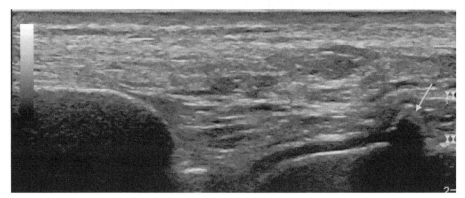

(B)

FIGURE 10.4 Sonograms demonstrating examples of bony irregularities. The image in (A) demonstrates an olecranon spur at the insertion of the triceps brachii (yellow arrow). The image in (B) shows an osteophyte on the talar dome at the tibial–talar joint.

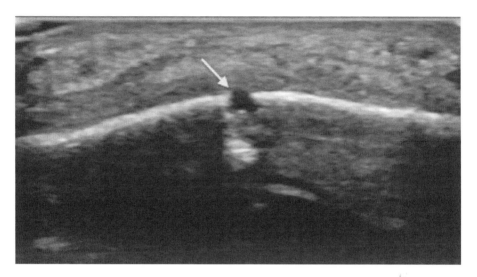

FIGURE 10.5 Sonogram demonstrating a cortical break in an individual with a nondisplaced fibular fracture.

Bone erosions and hypertrophy of the surrounding synovium with inflammation can be detected in inflammatory arthropathies with ultrasound. Increased Doppler uptake can reflect the surrounding inflammation (Figure 10.6).

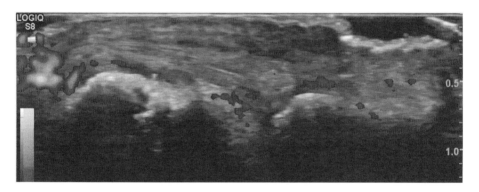

FIGURE 10.6 Sonogram demonstrating bony irregularity, erosions, and synovial inflammation seen as increased Doppler uptake in a patient with rheumatoid arthritis.

SKIN

The skin layer can be visualized with ultrasound. Detailed evaluation of the skin is not usually performed in a routine musculoskeletal evaluation; however, recognition of the skin layer is needed for appropriate localization of other structures. The skin varies in thickness between 1.4 and 4.8 mm depending on the location in the body. It consists of a superficial layer (the dermis) and a deep layer (epidermis). The skin is the most superficial layer of tissue seen in an ultrasound evaluation (Figure 10.7). For this reason, it is best appreciated with higher frequency transducers. Specialized transducers of very high frequency (20–50 MHz) are used for evaluation of dermatologic conditions. In a musculoskeletal assessment, disorders of normal skin such as infections, scar tissue, and tumors should be identified (Figure 10.8).

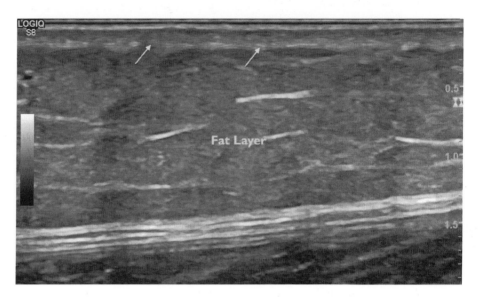

FIGURE 10.7 Sonogram demonstrating the skin (yellow arrows) and deeper subcutaneous layer containing fat.

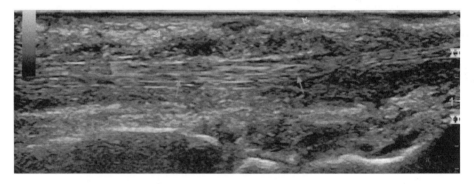

FIGURE 10.8 Sonogram demonstrating an alteration in the normal echotexture of skin. In this case, the heterogeneous postsurgical scar (yellow arrows) is shown. Note that the scar creates some mass effect on the underlying tendon (blue arrows).

FAT

Fat or adipose tissue is found as a part of the subcutaneous tissue and forms a protective layer over the deep musculoskeletal system. The fat layer is generally more hypoechoic than the surrounding tissue and should be identified to distinguish it from the surrounding tissue. The fat and subcutaneous layer is identified as hypoechoic lobules surrounded by hyperechoic septa (Figure 10.9). The subcutaneous layer also contains superficial veins and superficial nerves (Figure 10.10). The fat layer can be precisely measured with ultrasound. This can be of value when investigating fat atrophy, a known complication of steroid injections. Of note, deep areas of fat require lower frequencies of the incident sound waves for adequate penetration. For this reason, resolution of some of the deeper structures is reduced in patients with high body mass indexes.

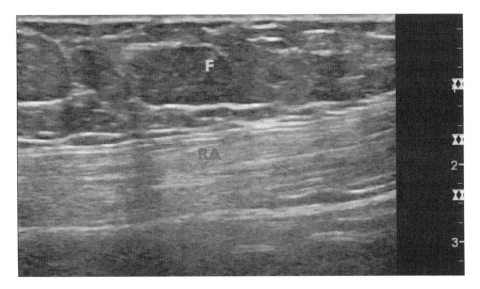

FIGURE 10.9 Sonogram showing the hypoechoic globular appearance of fat (F) in the subcutaneous layer. Note the more hyperechoic muscle layer (rectus abdominus [RA]) deep to the fat.

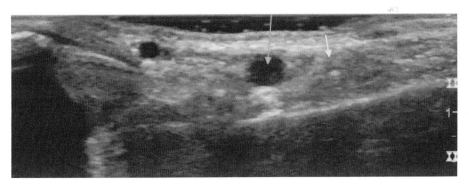

FIGURE 10.10 Sonogram of a short-axis view of the lesser saphenous vein (blue arrow) and the sural nerve (yellow arrow) in the subcutaneous tissue at the lateral ankle.

Areas of fat pads can be seen around long tendons (Figure 10.11) and should be examined for injury as they can be damaged along with other musculoskeletal structures (Figure 10.12). Trauma and fat necrosis can be identified by a loss of the normal echotexture of the lobules. Edema and infection such as cellulitis can also be identified in the subcutaneous layer with ultrasound. Edema presents as a hypoechoic signal between the lobules. With infection, there is a loss of the normal echotexture (Figure 10.13). Edema and cellulitis cannot always be reliably distinguished with ultrasound.

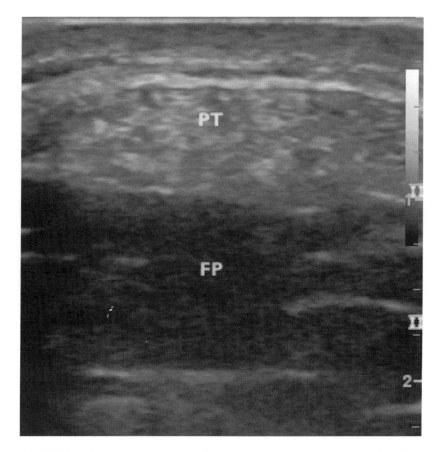

FIGURE 10.11 Sonogram demonstrating an example of a fat pad deep to a tendon. This image shows a short-axis view of the patellar tendon (PT) and deep to that is the fat pad of Hoffa (FP). Note the more hypoechoic appearance of the fat pad relative to the echotexture of the tendon.

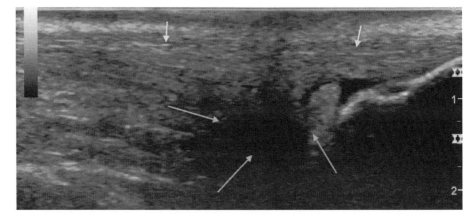

FIGURE 10.12 Sonogram demonstrating an example of pathology in an underlying fat pad. In this image, there is disruption of the normal echotexture of Kager's fat pad (blue arrows) anterior to the Achilles tendon (yellow arrows) suggesting abnormal edema from advanced Achilles tendonopathy.

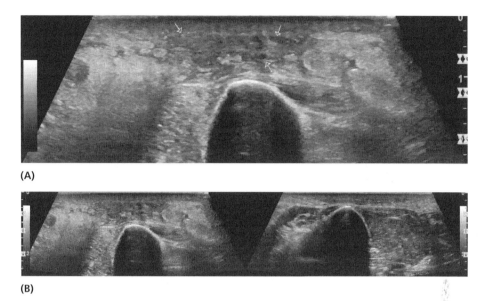

(A)

(B)

FIGURE 10.13 Sonograms demonstrating an appearance of cellulitis in the subcutaneous layer in a short-axis view of the forearm. The image in (A) shows a disruption of the echotexture and enlargement of the tissue (yellow arrows). The image in (B) shows the contrast between the affected limb (image on the left) and unaffected limb (image on the right).

CARTILAGE

In ultrasound imaging, cartilage is dark if it is fluid filled, and bright if it is not. Normal hyaline cartilage that covers smooth bony surfaces in joints is seen as a hypoechoic thin layer (Figure 10.14). By contrast, fibrocartilage such as the glenoid labrum or meniscus of the knee appears more hyperechoic (Figure 10.15). Fibrocartilage contains a large amount of collagen fibers that are highly reflective. Hyaline cartilage can be measured precisely with ultrasound for thinning. Fibrocartilage injuries typically appear as tears away from the bone or joint capsule.

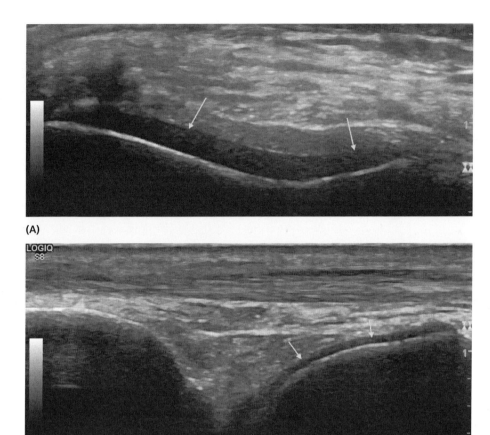

(A)

(B)

FIGURE 10.14 Sonograms demonstrating the hypoechoic hyaline cartilage at the knee (A) and the tibial–talar joint (B). Note how the cartilage follows the contour of the bone.

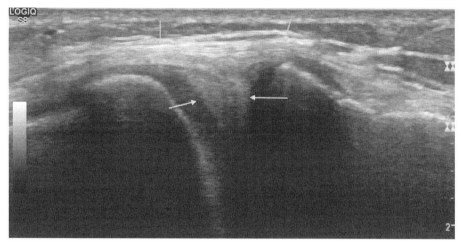

(A)

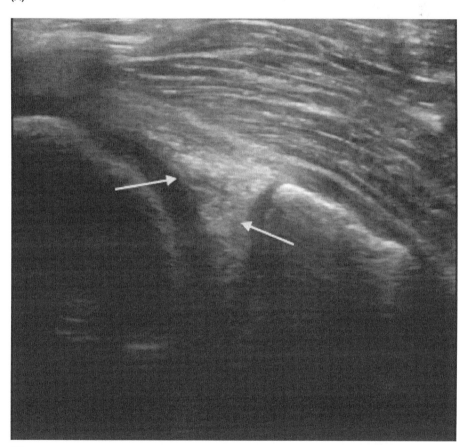

(B)

FIGURE 10.15 Sonograms demonstrating an example of the echogenic appearance of fibrocartilage. The images shown include the medial meniscus anterior horn (A) and posterior horn (B) (yellow arrows). Note that the appearance is hyperechoic in stark contrast to the hypoechoic appearance of hyaline cartilage. Also shown is the fibrillar pattern of the medial collateral ligament (A) (blue arrows).

LIGAMENTS

Ligaments have a moderately hyperechoic fibrillar appearance (Figures 10.15 and 10.16). Ligaments are most easily localized by placing the transducer between the bony landmarks that they connect. Like tendons, ligaments have a high degree of anisotropy, and the transducer should be positioned such that the incident sound waves are perpendicular to the path of the ligament. Anisotropic artifact could potentially be confused with ligament injury.

Ligaments will be found deep compared to the surrounding tendons. Stress maneuvers can be used to assess for integrity (Figure 10.17). Ligament injury can be reflected by irregularity of the fibrillar architecture or even complete disruption.

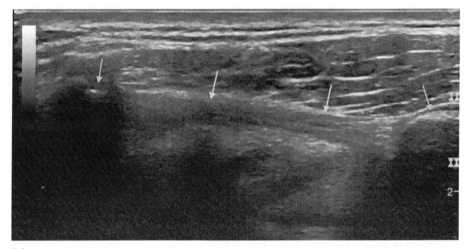

(A)

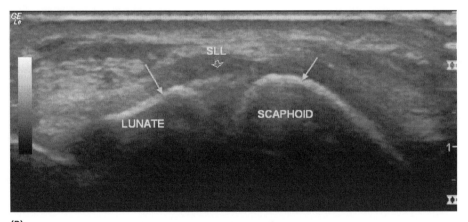

(B)

FIGURE 10.16 Sonograms demonstrating long-axis views of the fibrillar pattern of ligaments. The coracoacromial ligament (yellow arrows) is shown in (A) and the scapholunate ligament (SLL) (yellow arrow) is shown in (B). It is best to inspect a ligament by also visualizing the bony landmarks (blue arrows) that they attach.

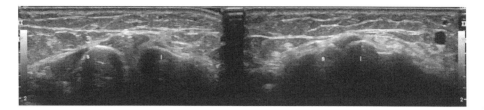

FIGURE 10.17 Sonogram demonstrating a split screen view of a normal scapholunate ligament (image on the right) in contrast to the injured side (image on the left) (s, scaphoid; l, lunate). Note that there is an abnormal widening of the joint space with stressing on the injured side.

BURSAE

A bursa is a synovial-lined sac that reduces friction between tissues such has tendon, bone, and muscle. Bursae are often only seen as potential spaces (Figure 10.18). For this reason, they are often difficult to visualize on ultrasound unless they are enlarged as in bursitis (Figure 10.19). Enlarged bursa should also be inspected for signs of calcification. Enlargement can be the result of excessive friction, direct trauma, or even infection. The findings of bursal enlargement should always be considered in the clinical context.

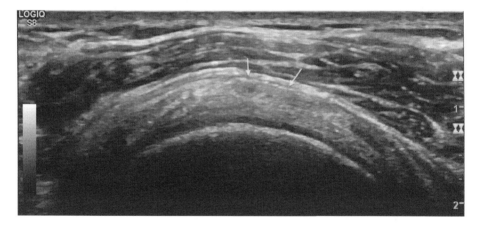

FIGURE 10.18 Sonogram demonstrating a normal appearance of the subacromial–subdeltoid bursa (yellow arrows). In normal conditions, this bursa is essentially seen as a potential space.

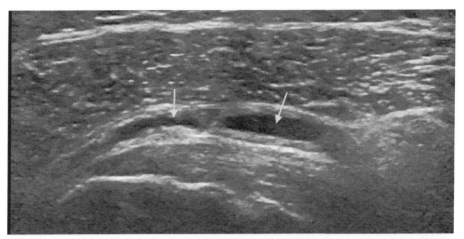

(A)

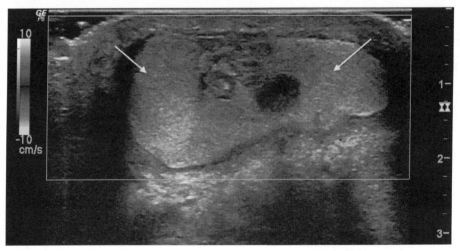

(B)

FIGURE 10.19 Sonograms demonstrating examples of abnormally enlarged bursa. The image in (A) shows an enlargement subacromial–subdeltoid bursitis (yellow arrows). The image in (B) shows a complex olecranon bursitis. Note that the complex bursitis does not appear as a simple anechoic enlargement and further investigation should be considered in the appropriate clinical context.

Bursae are classified according to location. Mucosal bursae lie between skin and bony prominences. Synovial bursae generally lie deeper and between muscle or tendon and bone. Bursae can also be classified as communicating or noncommunicating. They are considered communicating if the fluid is in continuity with the joint space. It is critical to learn the locations of clinically relevant bursa for a complete musculoskeletal inspection.

ARTERIES

Arteries are circular hypoechoic structures in short axis on ultra-sound and can be recognized by their pulsations. Increasing transducer pressure will cause the surrounding veins to col-lapse and often make the arterial pulsations more conspicu-ous (Figure 10.20). Doppler imaging provides further details. Color Doppler is generally preferable for higher flow ves-sels and power Doppler has higher sensitivity for lower flow states (Figure 10.21). Arteries should be viewed in both short and long axis for complete perspective (Figure 10.22). Arterial

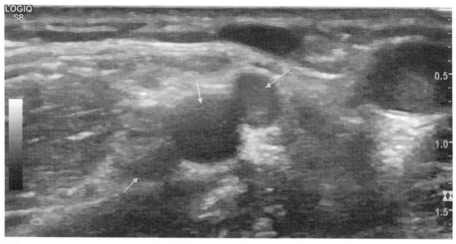

(A)

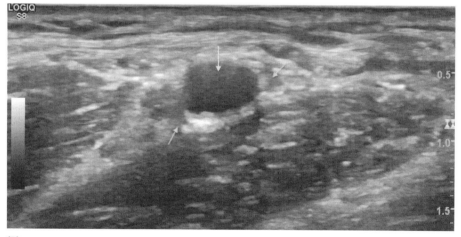

(B)

FIGURE 10.20 Sonograms demonstrating short-axis views of the brachial artery (yellow arrows) and surrounding veins (blue arrows). The veins are evident in (A) with less transducer pressure. They are collapsed in (B) due to more transducer pressure.

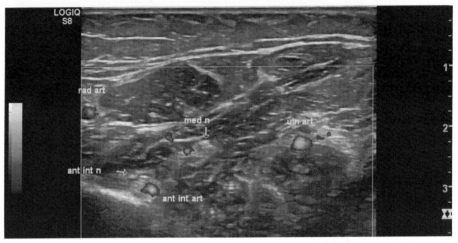

(A)

(B)

FIGURE 10.21 Sonograms demonstrating short-axis views of arteries with color Doppler (A) and power Doppler (B). The image in (A) shows the brachial artery. Color Doppler generally provides a better assessment of higher flow states. It also provides information on the direction of flow in relation to the transducer. The image in (B) is a cross-sectional view of the mid-forearm. The power Doppler in this image provides visualization of the major arteries including some of the smaller ones. The arteries shown include the radial artery (rad art), ulnar artery (uln art), anterior interosseus artery (ant int art), and the persistent median artery (not labeled, near the median nerve [med n]). Power Doppler is often preferable for its higher sensitivity to some of the smaller arteries.

injuries, including aneurysms and pseudoaneuryms, can often be detected with ultrasound and the use of Doppler imaging can help to distinguish them from other masses (Figure 10.23).

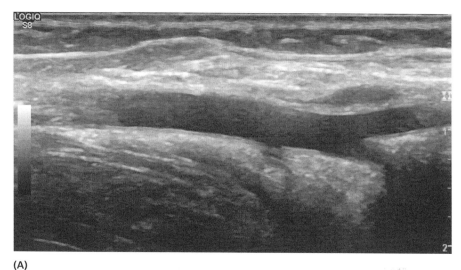

(A)

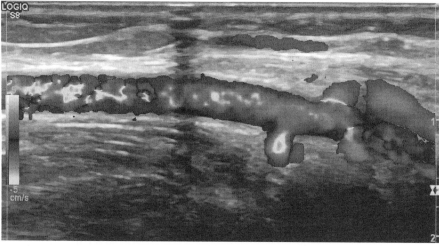

(B)

FIGURE 10.22 Sonograms of a long-axis view of the brachial artery with both conventional gray scale (A) and color Doppler (B) imaging. The long-axis view provides an additional perspective with flow, arterial branches, and surrounding tissue.

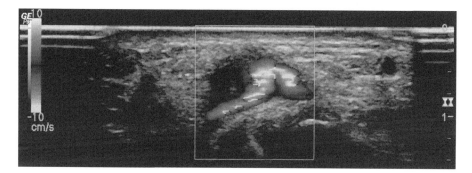

FIGURE 10.23 Sonogram of a palpable mass identified as a radial artery pseudoaneurysm with color Doppler ultrasound.

VEINS

Veins can be easily distinguished from arteries by their compressibility (Figure 10.24). For this reason, the examiner should use only light pressure when first attempting to identify a vein. Blood flow can be seen through veins with color or power Doppler. Veins lack the constant flow with Doppler imaging, which is characteristic of arteries. Flow can be accentuated with compression and decompression of a vein (Figure 10.25). Similar to arteries, veins should be assessed in both short and long axis (Figure 10.26). The long-axis view is generally more reliable when assessing the compressibility of a vein (Figure 10.27). Lack of normal compressibility suggests the likelihood of venous thrombosis. The loss of anechoic appearance and loss of flow in the vein are additional suggestions of thrombosis (Figure 10.28). Because of the implications, it should also be determined whether the thrombosis is within a deep or superficial vein (Figure 10.29). The patient should be referred for a conventional venous Doppler evaluation if deep venous thrombosis is suspected during a musculoskeletal evaluation, particularly if the practitioner is not experienced in the diagnosis of vascular conditions.

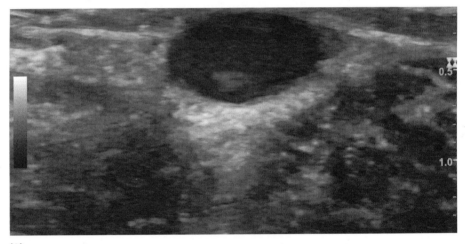

(A)

FIGURE 10.24 Sonograms demonstrating a short-axis view of the effect of transducer pressure on the appearance of a vein. Figures (A) through (E) show progressively increasing pressure.

(continued)

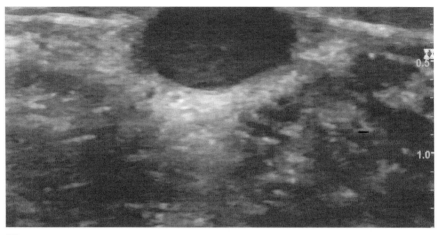

(B)

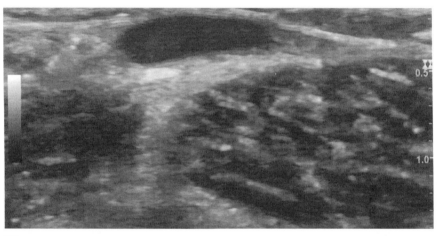

(C)

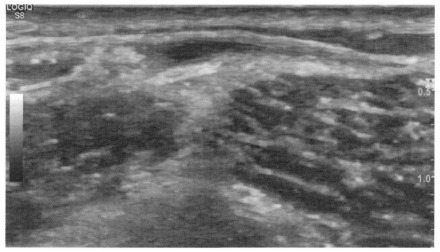

(D)

FIGURE 10.24 *(continued)*

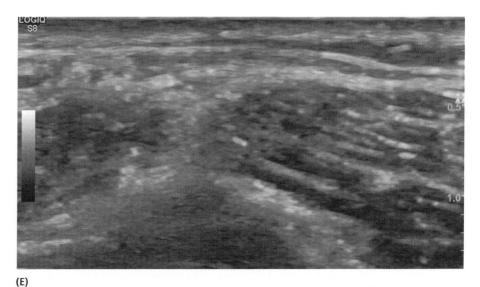

(E)

FIGURE 10.24 (*continued*)

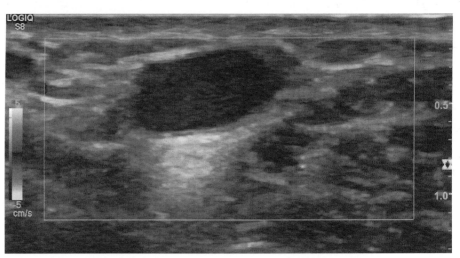

(A)

FIGURE 10.25 Sonograms demonstrating a short-axis view of a vein with color Doppler both before (A) and after (B) compression and release with the accentuation of flow. Care should be taken while assessing the nature of the Doppler flow to avoid confusion with an artery.

(*continued*)

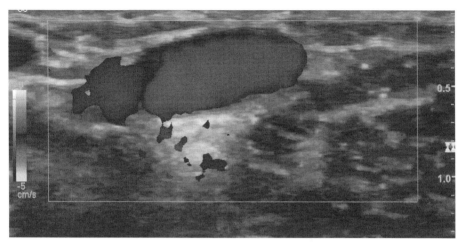

(B)

FIGURE 10.25 (*continued*)

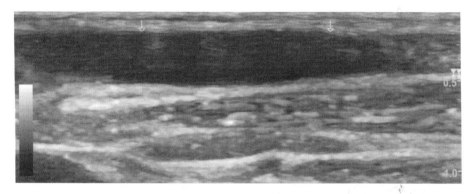

FIGURE 10.26 Sonogram showing a long-axis view of a vein.

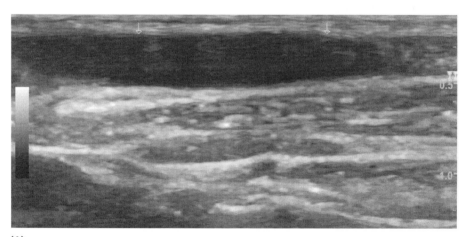

(A)

FIGURE 10.27 Sonograms demonstrating a long-axis view of the effect of pressure on a vein. The images (A) through (D) are with progressively increasing transducer pressure. This degree of compressibility is characteristic of a normal vein.

(*continued*)

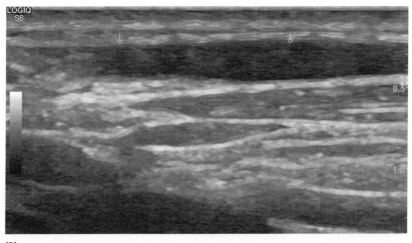

(B)

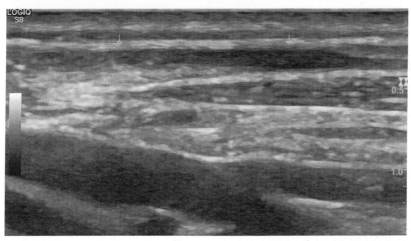

(C)

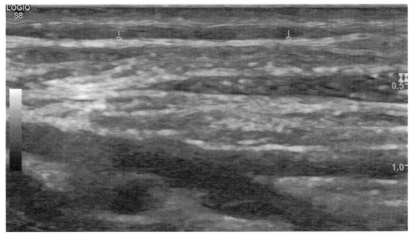

(D)

FIGURE 10.27 (*continued*)

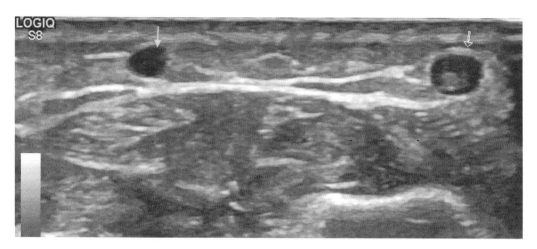

FIGURE 10.28 Sonogram demonstrating a short-axis view of a superficial venous thrombosis (yellow arrow) in contrast to an unaffected vein (blue arrow). The more hyperechoic thrombosis can be seen obstructing the anechoic lumen.

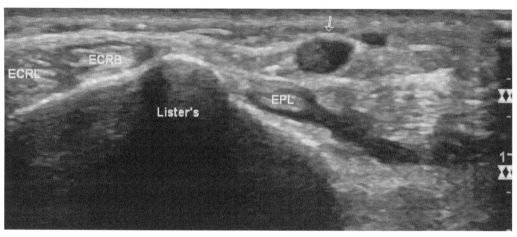

(A)

FIGURE 10.29 Sonograms demonstrating short-axis views of examples of relatively small superficial (A) and deep (B) venous thrombosis (yellow arrows). The image in (A) shows the partial obstruction of the anechoic lumen of a superficial vein at the left of the dorsal wrist. It is distinguished from other anatomic landmarks at that level, including the extensor carpi radialis longus (ECRL), extensor carpi radialis brevis (ECRB), and extensor pollicis longus (EPL) tendons as well as the bony landmark of Lister's tubercle. The image in (B) shows enlargement and occlusion of the veins (yellow arrows) in the medial gastrocnemius reflected in the complete loss of anechoic appearance. The discovery of thrombosis in the deep veins requires consideration of medical intervention for possible anticoagulation therapy.

(continued)

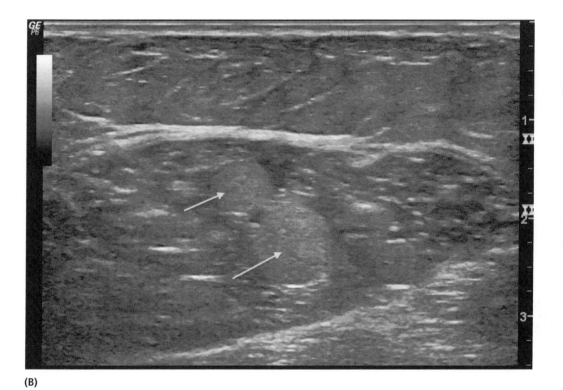

(B)

FIGURE 10.29 (*continued*)

REMEMBER

1) Bony landmarks serve as some of the best structures to maintain orientation to the surrounding anatomy.
2) Use the highest resolution available to evaluate very superficial tissue such as skin.
3) Evaluate the surrounding fat pads of musculoskeletal structures for additional clues to potential injury.
4) Hyaline cartilage has a hypoechoic appearance on ultrasound whereas fibrocartilage appears hyperechoic.
5) Localize ligaments by finding the acoustic landmarks of their bony attachments.
6) Study the clinically relevant bursa and develop a detailed knowledge of their anatomic location.
7) Analyze arteries and veins in both short and long axis and include Doppler imaging.

BIBLIOGRAPHY

1. Bianchi S, Martinoli C, eds. *Ultrasound of the Musculoskeletal System.* Berlin, Germany: Springer-Verlag; 2007.

2. Fornage BD, Deshayes JL. Ultrasound of normal skin. *J Clin Ultrasound.* 1986;14(8):619-622.

3. Jacobson JA. *Fundamentals of Musculoskeletal Ultrasound.* 2nd ed. Philadelphia, PA: Elsevier Saunders; 2013.

4. Resnick D. *Diagnosis of Bone and Joint Disorders.* 3rd ed. Philadelphia, PA: W.B. Saunders; 1995.

5. Smith J, Finnoff JT. Diagnostic and interventional musculoskeletal ultrasound: part 1. Fundamentals. *PM & R.* 2009;1(1):64-75.

6. Strakowski JA. *Ultrasound Evaluation of Focal Neuropathies. Correlation With Electrodiagnosis.* New York, NY: Demos Medical; 2014.

7. Van Holsbeeck MT, Introcaso JS. *Musculoskeletal Ultrasound.* 2nd ed. St. Louis, MO: Mosby; 2001.

Imaging Masses

A systematic approach to masses is needed for anyone involved in musculoskeletal ultrasound. They can be encountered incidentally in routine examinations and frequently are the presenting complaint. A tissue diagnosis cannot be reliably determined on every ultrasound examination, but characteristic features can be distinguished that are often helpful for determination of the need for additional evaluation as well as management decisions. Some of these features include the size, nature of the border, echotexture, compressibility, relationship to surrounding tissue, and relative vascularity.

DETERMINING SIZE

Ultrasound is an excellent modality for measuring the size of a mass. Most ultrasound instruments can provide measurements that are accurate within fractions of a millimeter. Masses should be scanned in both short- and long-axis planes. It is typical to report the linear measurement of three orthogonal planes, referred by some as maximum length, width, and height (Figure 11.1). Care should be used to completely scan and identify the entirety of the mass. In cases in which the mass displays an irregular shape or border, and these parameters are difficult to reliably determine, this shape should be described and the relative size should be reported to the extent possible (Figure 11.2). Ultrasound also is an excellent, cost-effective modality for following progression of mass size, shape, and other characteristic changes over time.

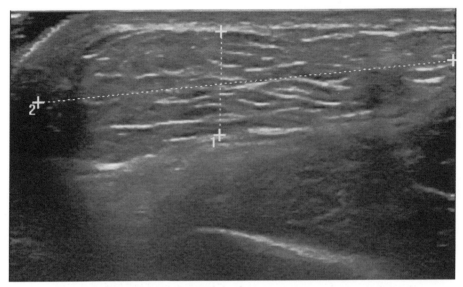

(A)

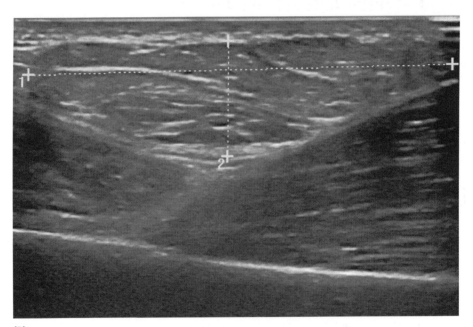

(B)

FIGURE 11.1 Sonograms demonstrating short-axis view (A) and long-axis view (B) of a superficial mass (lipoma) demonstrating use of linear measurement to assess the size. The length and width are obtained using the two views. The depth should be consistent between the two views. Note the difference in echotexture between the mass and both the superficial dermal layer and deeper muscle layer.

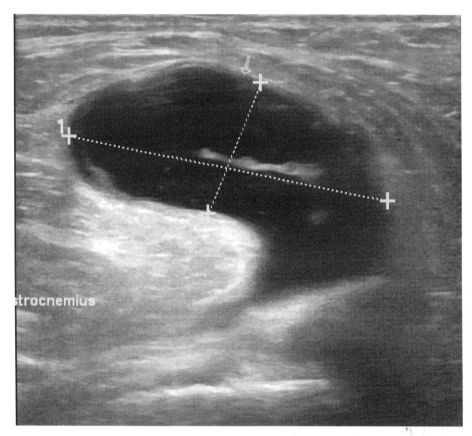

FIGURE 11.2 Sonogram of an irregularly shaped mass (semimembranosus-medial gastrocnemius [Baker's] cyst) that limits the precision of size determination with linear measurements. In such cases, the size is reported to the extent possible and the shape and other characteristics are included in the description.

NATURE OF THE BORDER

The characteristics of the border of masses often provide important clues of their nature and should be reported in the medical record. Masses with irregular borders often have different implications than those with smooth borders with well-defined walls (Figure 11.3). It should be noted when the mass appears contiguous with the surrounding tissue as opposed to having well-defined borders. The overall shape of the mass should also be considered and described.

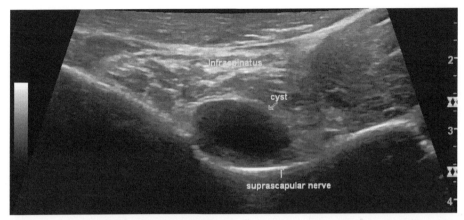

(A)

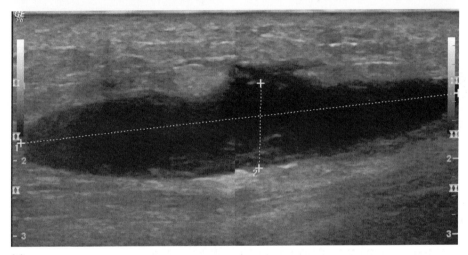

(B)

FIGURE 11.3 Sonograms demonstrating examples of different borders of otherwise similar appearing masses. The image in (A) displays a mass (cyst) with well-defined walls. The image in (B) has a similar echogenic appearance as the cyst but does not have a well-defined border over its entire circumference. This image represents a hematoma that lies within a fascial plane. Some of the fluid infiltrates the overlying tissue in an irregular pattern as a clue that it is not cystic. Note that this image is a split-screen approximation used to visualize the length in one picture. Additional consideration should be given to the location of the mass in relation to other tissue. Note that the cyst in image (A) is in proximity to the suprascapular nerve creating neuropathy as a result of mass effect.

ECHOTEXTURE

The nature of the echotexture of the mass should be considered. It should be described in relation to the surrounding tissue but also in reference to its own relative uniformity. The mass should be defined as hypo, hyper, or isoechoic relative to the structures around it (Figure 11.4). The echotexture can help determine if the mass is cystic or solid. The presence of any septations or divisions within the mass should also be noted (Figure 11.5).

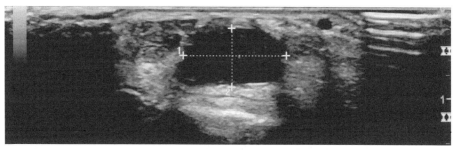

(A)

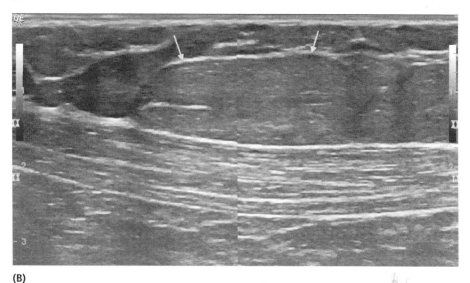

(B)

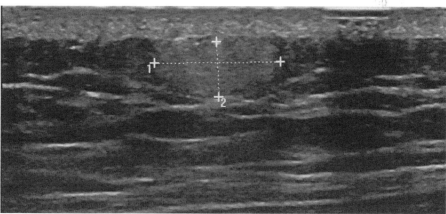

(C)

FIGURE 11.4 Sonograms demonstrating examples of masses with different echotextures. In (A), the mass is hypoechoic relative to the surrounding tissue. This particular mass is a ganglion cyst. In (B), the mass is relatively isoechoic relative to the surrounding subcutaneous tissue. This mass is a lipoma with echotexture similar to the surrounding adipose. Note that the echotexture is distinct from the underlying muscle layer. In (C), the mass is hyperechoic relative to the surrounding tissue. A mass with this echotexture often might require biopsy or excision for a specific tissue diagnosis.

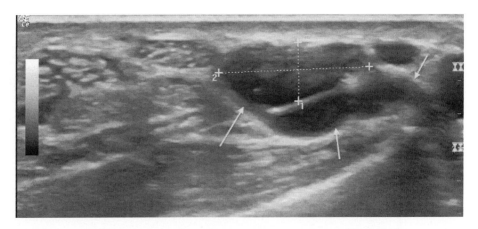

FIGURE 11.5 Sonogram demonstrating a mass (ganglion cyst) with multiple septations (yellow arrows).

COMPRESSIBILITY

The relative compressibility of a mass can be determined by the amount of pressure exerted by the transducer. There is deformation of most soft tissue with increasing transducer pressure (Figure 5.3) but the extent of change of the mass relative to the surrounding structures can often be helpful. A cyst or vascular structure will typically deform with external pressure to a much greater extent than a solid mass.

POSITIONAL RELATIONSHIP TO SURROUNDING TISSUE

The location of the mass in relationship to other anatomic structures should be determined and reported as it can be a valuable clue toward determining the nature of the mass as well as its potential complications from occupying space. The proximity to tendons, joint spaces, and neurovascular bundles should be of particular emphasis. Any displacement of surrounding tissue should be identified [Figures 11.3(A) and 11.6]. It should be noted when the mass is infiltrating other tissue, which is more typical in malignant conditions.

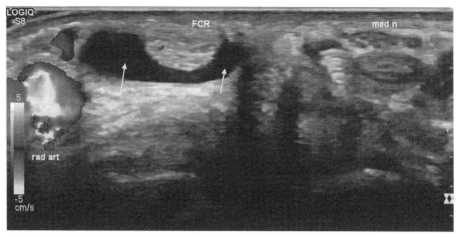

(A)

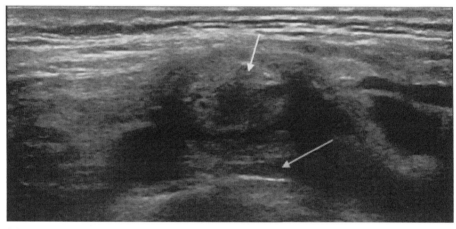

(B)

FIGURE 11.6 Sonograms demonstrating examples of mass effect on surrounding tissue from the mass. The image in (A) shows a short-axis view of a ganglion (yellow arrows) causing compression and discomfort on the distal flexor carpi radialis (FCR) tendon. Note also the location of the radial artery (rad art) and median nerve (med n). The image in (B) shows a view of a solid supraclavicular mass (yellow arrow) causing compression of the subclavian vein (blue arrow). Understanding the relationship of the mass to the surrounding tissue can sometimes provide insight into the patient's clinical condition.

RELATIVE VASCULARITY

Use of Doppler imaging is helpful for assessing the relative vascularity of a mass (Figure 11.7). Color Doppler is generally more effective for higher flow states and Power Doppler for identifying smaller vessels (see Chapter 6). Efforts should be made to distinguish if any vascularity is within the mass or external to it. Vascularity of a mass is more frequently seen with malignant conditions. This is not always a reliable parameter for distinguishing a benign from a malignant mass. Other imaging modalities and biopsy or referral for excision should be considered when further investigation is warranted.

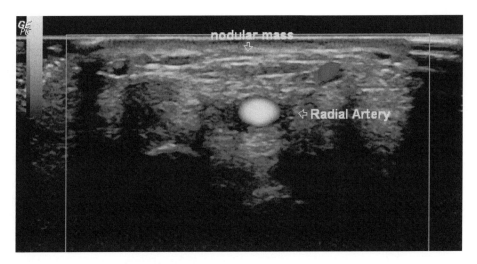

FIGURE 11.7 Sonogram demonstrating the use of Doppler imaging to assess the relative vascularity of a palpable mass. In this image, there are no signs of vascularity intrinsic to the mass but only extrinsic.

REMEMBER ·

1) When assessing a mass, determine whether it is solid or cystic and whether the border is smooth or irregular.
2) Measure the size of the mass using the measurement tools on the ultrasound machine and use three orthogonal planes.
3) Determine if the mass invades surrounding tissue.
4) Use Doppler imaging to assess the vascularity of the mass.
5) Do not attempt to make a tissue diagnosis of the mass, particularly when inexperienced. Refer to other imaging modalities such as MRI and other assessment when appropriate.

BIBLIOGRAPHY

1. Bianchi S, Martinoli C. *Ultrasound of the Musculoskeletal System*. Heidelberg: Springer-Verlag; 2007.

2. Enzinger FM, Weiss SW. *Soft Tissue Tumors*. 3rd ed. St. Louis, MO: Mosby; 1995:821–928.

3. Jacobson JA. *Fundamentals of Musculoskeletal Ultrasound*. 2nd ed. Philadelphia, PA: Elsevier Saunders; 2013.

4. Van Holsbeeck MT, Introcaso JS. *Musculoskeletal Ultrasound*. 2nd ed. St. Louis, MO: Mosby; 2001.

12

Foreign Bodies

INTRODUCTION

Identification and removal of foreign bodies can be extremely challenging in some circumstances. Plain film radiography has traditionally been the imaging modality of choice for most foreign bodies. Foreign bodies that are not radiopaque are not visualized by these methods. Ultrasound is an excellent modality for identifying foreign bodies. It has high resolution and can frequently be used to identify the nature of the foreign body by the echotexture and surrounding artifact. It is also excellent for identifying the effect of the foreign body on the surrounding tissue. Ultrasound is also the ideal imaging modality for dynamic guidance for removal of the foreign body.

Identifying the size and relationship to other tissue can provide useful information prior to removal. Precise localization helps to minimize any surgical exploration or improve the approach to percutaneous removal (Figure 12.1). Most foreign bodies are hyperechoic with a hypoechoic ring of reactive tissue around it (Figure 12.2). Reverberation artifact is typical for foreign bodies and aids in detection (Figure 12.3). The posterior artifact tends to become larger and more irregular with larger foreign bodies. Reverberation artifact is discussed in more detail in Chapter 13. Detecting surrounding inflammation or infection also provides valuable information for the clinical approach (Figure 12.4).

Detailed discussion of the nature of various foreign bodies is beyond the scope of this text. Metal, wood, and glass are some of the most commonly encountered foreign bodies and have some distinguishing characteristics.

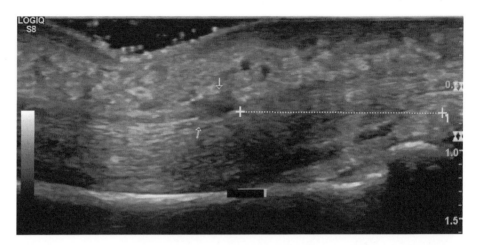

FIGURE 12.1 Sonogram demonstrating an example of precise localization of a foreign body (yellow arrows) just superficial to the flexor digitorum profundus tendon. The linear measurement is used to provide precise distance from the midportion of the proximal interphalangeal joint.

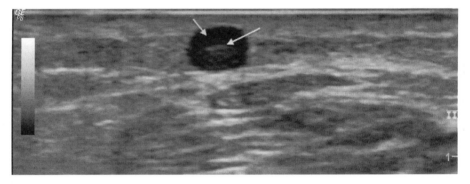

FIGURE 12.2 Sonogram demonstrating a relatively hyperechoic foreign body (yellow arrow) with an anechoic ring of reactive fluid around it (blue arrow).

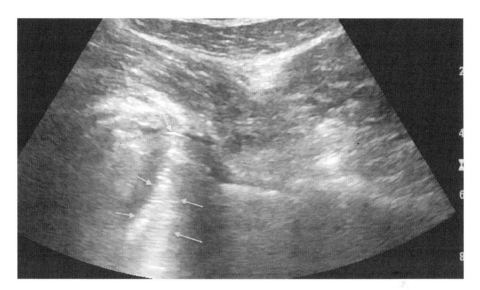

FIGURE 12.3 Sonogram demonstrating reverberation artifact (blue arrows) deep to metal artifact (yellow arrow). Reverberation artifact occurs when the sound waves bounce between two interfaces with very high impedance, such as foreign bodies.

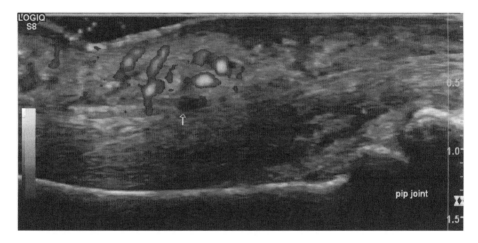

FIGURE 12.4 Sonogram demonstrating significant inflammatory reaction with increased Doppler signal around a foreign body (yellow arrow).

METAL

Metal appears hyperechoic and tends to have the most reverberation artifact of the foreign bodies (Figure 12.5).

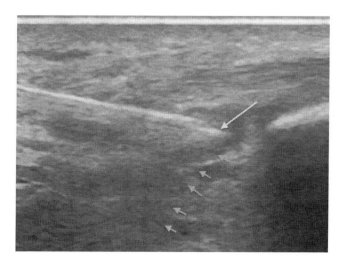

FIGURE 12.5 Sonogram demonstrating the reverberation artifact seen with metal as a foreign body. The tip of the needle is shown (yellow arrow) with the reverberation artifact deep to that (blue arrows).

WOOD

Wood initially appears hyperechoic but tends to become more hypoechoic over time. The foreign body itself can become somewhat less conspicuous, however, the reactive tissue around it tends to become more prominent. Wood tends to have a fairly large amount of posterior shadowing (Figure 12.6).

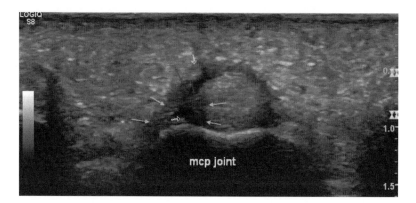

FIGURE 12.6 Sonogram demonstrating the appearance of a small wood splinter (red arrow) positioned against the flexor digitorum profundus and superficialis tendons (seen in short axis). Both reactive tissue edema (yellow arrows) is seen as well as posterior shadowing (blue arrows). In this case, the splinter had been present for many weeks and note that the wooden foreign body itself is relatively hypoechoic.

GLASS

Glass generally appears hyperechoic with a relatively small amount of posterior reverberation (Figure 12.7).

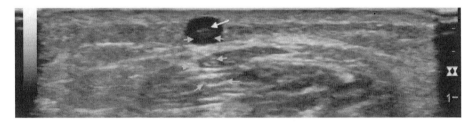

FIGURE 12.7 Sonogram demonstrating the appearance of a small sliver of glass (yellow arrow). Note that there is a combination of a small degree of reverberation artifact and shadowing (blue arrows). The reverberation artifact (seen best just beneath the glass sliver within the anechoic circle) is much less than is seen with metal. The posterior shadowing is significantly less than typically seen with wood.

Ultrasound can be used to assist with needle guidance when percutaneous removal of the foreign body is desired. This allows simultaneous visualization of the needle and foreign body in real time. It is generally best to approach this procedure with the needle in-plane with respect to the orientation of the transducer. See Chapter 14 for a detailed discussion on needle guidance with ultrasound.

REMEMBER ···

1) It is helpful to not only assess the appearance of the foreign body, but also the extent of the surrounding tissue reaction and the degree and nature of the posterior artifact.
2) Precise localization and measurement of the foreign body should be performed to maximize the ease of removal.
3) Use Doppler imaging to assess the degree of inflammation, and also consider the possibility of infection.

BIBLIOGRAPHY

1. Horton LK, Jacobson JA, Powell A, et al. Sonography and radiography of soft-tissue foreign bodies. *AJR Am J Roentgenol*. 2001;176(5):1155–1159.

2. Jacobson JA. *Fundamentals of Musculoskeletal Ultrasound*. 2nd ed. Philadelphia, PA: Elsevier Saunders; 2013.

3. Saboo SS, Saboo SH, Soni SS, Adhane V. High-resolution sonography is effective in detection of soft tissue foreign bodies: experience from a rural Indian center. *J Ultrasound Med*. 2009;28(9):1245–1249.

4. Shrestha D, Sharma UK, Mohammad R, Dhoju D. The role of ultrasonography in detection and localization of radiolucent foreign body in soft tissues of extremities. *JNMA J Nepal Med Assoc*. 2009;48(173):5–9.

CHAPTER 13

Artifacts

Artifacts in musculoskeletal ultrasound refer to features in the ultrasound image that do not reliably represent the anatomic structure underneath the transducer. Knowledge of artifacts is critical for reliably interpreting images in musculoskeletal ultrasound. Some artifacts such as anisotropy can be minimized with appropriate scanning technique. Others must be simply recognized for appropriate image interpretation. Artifacts can even provide clinical clues for underlying pathology in some circumstances. A detailed discussion of all of the potential artifacts that can be encountered with ultrasound is beyond the scope of this text; however, the more common ones are mentioned.

ANISOTROPY

Anisotropy is the most significant and commonly encountered artifact with the superficial structures in musculoskeletal ultrasound and it is particularly potentially problematic when using linear transducers. It refers to the property of tissue to differentially conduct or reflect sound waves back to the transducer based on the angle of incidence of the sound waves. Anisotropic artifact refers to a darkening and loss of resolution of the image (Figures 4.7 and 13.1). This occurs when the approach of the sound waves is less than perpendicular (ie, angle of incidence greater than 0 degrees) (Figure 2.7). Therefore, the examiner should attempt to keep the direction of the beam as close to perpendicular as possible.

Tendons are particularly prone to anisotropic artifact due to their high reflectivity and uniform linear orientation (Figure 9.10) (see Chapter 7). Most other tissues have a degree of anisotropy. Conspicuity of a needle is also affected by anisotropy. Effort should be made to maintain the incident sound wave as close to perpendicular to the needle as possible. This is discussed in more detail in Chapter 14. Techniques such as toggling the transducer and heel-to-toe rocking should be used to reduce anisotropy. These maneuvers are discussed in Chapter 5.

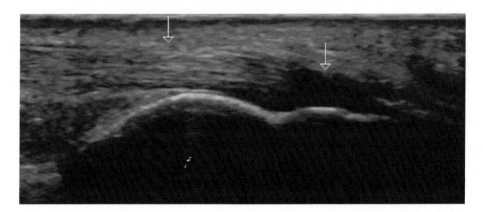

FIGURE 13.1 Sonogram demonstrating an example of signal change due to anisotropic artifact. The image displays a long-axis view of a normal Achilles tendon with insertion on the calcaneus. The yellow arrows represent the direction of the approaching sound waves from the transducer. The normal fibrillar architecture of the tendon is seen toward the left of the screen where the angle of incidence is orthogonal to the tendon. Note the hypoechoic appearance of the tendon fibers as they curve at a steep angle to insert into the calcaneus. This is anisotropic artifact related to this portion of the tendon not being perpendicular to the incident sound beam. This artifact can be resolved by performing a heel-to-toe rock with the transducer to change the angle of incidence to the distal portion. Failure to recognize the effect of anisotropy on an image like this could lead to an erroneous conclusion of pathology.

INADEQUATE CONDUCTION MEDIUM

Ultrasonography requires a sufficient amount of conduction median between the transducer and the skin of the patient for the sound waves to adequately travel from the transducer to the tissue and back to provide a clear image. This is usually done with conduction gel (Figure 13.2) or less frequently stand-off pads. This is necessary because ultrasound waves do not conduct well through air. They need a medium such as gels or liquid to create a good image. The examiner should use a liberal amount of conduction gel to avoid the artifact caused by a lack of effective sound wave transmission (Figure 13.3).

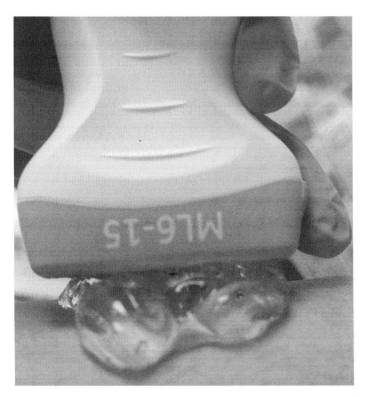

FIGURE 13.2 Picture demonstrating the use of conduction gel to enhance the transmission of sound waves between the tissue and the transducer.

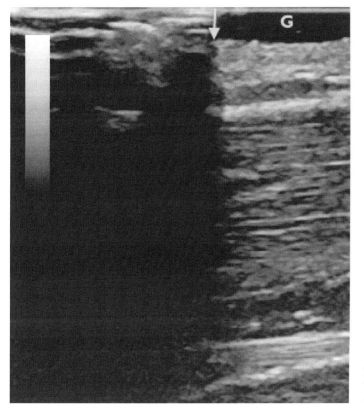

FIGURE 13.3 Sonogram demonstrating the effect of inadequate conduction gel on the ultrasound image. The tissue is relatively uniform superficial muscle. The right side of the image has gel under the transducer (the gel is the anechoic superficial region on the right side of the screen labeled G). Note that the tissue to the right of the yellow arrow is under the gel and clearly visible. The left darkened area is under the portion of the transducer without the gel. This impaired image results from the lack of sound wave transmission between the tissue and the transducer in the field where there is not an adequate conduction medium.

POSTERIOR ACOUSTIC SHADOWING

Posterior acoustic shadowing refers to a darkening of the ultrasound image beneath a structure with a large amount of reflectivity. Examples of this include decreased signal underneath tumors, calcifications, or foreign bodies (Figure 13.4). The tissue below an object of higher impedance receives less of the incident sound waves than surrounding tissue that is not below that object and appears darker. Surveying the entire ultrasound image rather than simply focusing a single structure can help to identify posterior acoustic shadowing by recognizing the darkening throughout the image in a vertical line. This artifact is sometimes more evident than the appearance

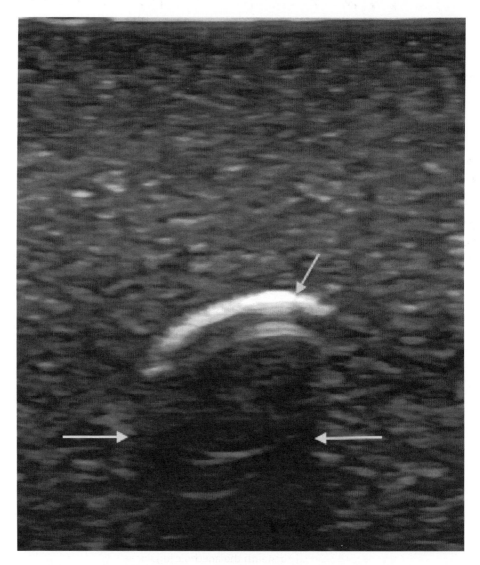

FIGURE 13.4 Sonogram demonstrating the effect of posterior acoustic shadowing (yellow arrows) beneath a highly reflective foreign body (blue arrow).

of the actual structure causing the posterior acoustic shadowing and can be used to help to identify the location of a tumor or foreign body.

POSTERIOR ACOUSTIC ENHANCEMENT

Posterior acoustic enhancement, also known as increased through transmission, occurs as a result of a focal area of decreased impedance that lead to an increased transmission of sound waves to the tissue immediately below it. It is essentially the reciprocal of posterior acoustic shadowing. Cysts and veins are examples of structures that can lead to posterior acoustic enhancement (Figure 13.5). Because a greater amount of sound waves return to the transducer from tissue with less impendence above it, that tissue generally appears more hyperechoic. If the source of artifact can be compressed such as a vein, increased transducer pressure can reduce or eliminate it. Similar to other artifacts, the entire image should be analyzed to recognize

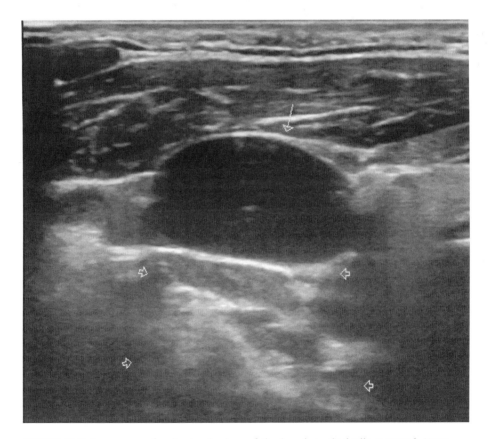

FIGURE 13.5 Sonogram of a short-axis view of the jugular vein (yellow arrow). Note that the tissue directly beneath the anechoic jugular vein (yellow arrowheads) is more hyperechoic than the tissue lateral to that. The effect is produced because the vein has less attenuation of the sound waves than the surrounding solid tissue.

the focal brightness seen throughout all of the tissue in a vertical line below the area of decreased impedance. In some circumstances, posterior acoustic enhancement can be used to provide clinical clues for assessment by enhancing conspicuity of underlying structures (Figure 13.6).

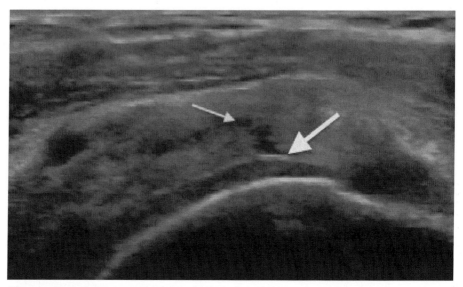

(A)

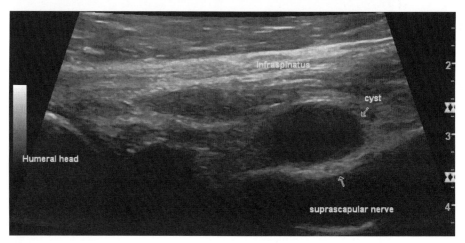

(B)

FIGURE 13.6 Sonograms demonstrating examples of posterior acoustic enhancement providing additional clinical clues. The image in (A) is a long-axis view of the supraspinatus tendon. In this image, the decrease in overlying tissue density as a result of the tendon tear (blue arrow) results in posterior acoustic enhancement and improved visualization of the border of the articular cartilage (yellow arrow). The enhancement of border of the cartilage is a clinical clue suggesting overlying rotator cuff tear, even in circumstances when the tear is less conspicuous. The image in (B) is a long-axis view of the infraspinatus tendon with a posterior labral cyst. This image shows good visualization of the suprascapular nerve that lies below the cyst. The nerve is often difficult to see with such clarity in ordinary circumstances.

REVERBERATION ARTIFACT

Reverberation artifact occurs as a result of repetitive reflection back and forth between two highly reflective surfaces (Figure 13.7). In musculoskeletal ultrasound, it is most frequently encountered with needle guidance and metallic implants (Figure 13.8). This artifact appears as equally spaced hyperechoic lines that blur the image. It is particularly important to recognize that this artifact makes the metallic structure appear thicker and deeper than it really is.

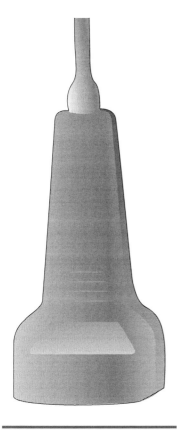

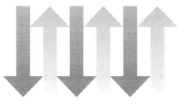

FIGURE 13.7 Illustration of the development of reverberation artifact. The sound waves bounce back and forth between a superficial object with high impendence and the transducer.

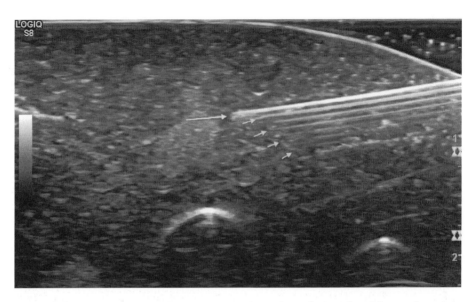

FIGURE 13.8 Sonogram demonstrating an in-plane view of a needle with reverberation artifact. The needle tip is identified by the position of the yellow arrow. The equally spaced hyperechoic artifact (blue arrows) is beneath the actual needle.

Other forms of specific descriptions of reverberation artifact include *comet-tail* and *ring-down* artifact. Comet tail artifact usually occurs because of reflection between two closely located structures. The tapering tail appearance results from attenuation of the artifact as it moves more deeply (Figure 13.9). Ring-down artifact looks similar, but is related to deep air pockets.

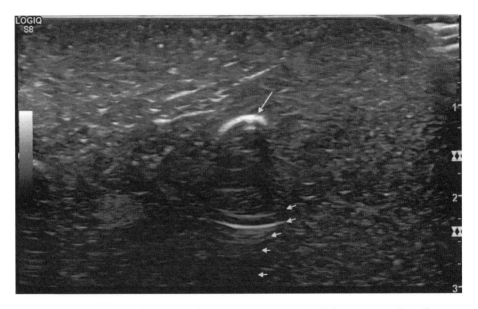

FIGURE 13.9 Sonogram demonstrating an appearance resembling comet tail artifact (blue arrows). The artifact lies beneath a highly reflective structure (yellow arrow) and tapers with attenuation as it extends deeper.

OTHER ARTIFACTS

There are many other types of artifacts seen with ultrasound and a detailed description is beyond the scope of this text. Many of them are related to variations in the signal between tissues of different densities. Ultrasound images are based on the assumption that sound waves are traveling through tissue at a relatively uniform speed (1,540 m/s in human tissue). Tissue variation with significantly different densities can potentially "fool" the instrumentation into creating an image that does not completely represent the anatomic structure. Excessive refraction and attenuation can also occur with tissues of differing densities. These types of artifacts more frequently are problematic in ultrasound of deeper structures as opposed to those typically viewed in a musculoskeletal evaluation.

REMEMBER ·

1) The entire screen of the ultrasound image should be assessed to help detect artifact.
2) The transducer should be positioned so that the direction of the incident sound waves is perpendicular to the tissue of interest to minimize anisotropic artifact.
3) Posterior acoustic enhancement can sometimes be used to provide clinical clues and increased conspicuity of tissue.

BIBLIOGRAPHY

1. Connolly D, Berman L, McNally E. The use of beam angulation to overcome anisotropy when viewing human tendon with high frequency linear array ultrasound. *Br J Radiol.* 2001;74:183–185.

2. Feldman MK, Katyal S, Blackwood MS. US artifacts. *Radiographics.* 2009;29:1179–1189.

3. Kremkau FW. *Diagnostic Ultrasound: Principles and Ultrasound.* St. Louis, MO: Saunders; 2002.

4. Rubin JM, Adler RS, Bude RO, et al. Clean and dirty shadowing at US: a reappraisal. *Radiology.* 1991;181:231–236.

5. Scanlon KA. Sonographic artifacts and their origins. *Am J Roentgenol.* 1991;156:1267–1272.

CHAPTER 14

Ultrasound Guidance for Injections

Ultrasound is the ideal imaging modality for guiding most peripheral joint, tendon, and nerve injections. It allows visualization of both the needle and soft tissue target in real time. This improves accuracy of needle placement for both injection and aspiration procedures and allows identification of neurovascular and other visceral structures for avoidance.

INDICATIONS FOR ULTRASOUND GUIDANCE

The use of ultrasound guidance for various injections is often a matter of debate. Some argue that it is unnecessary for many simple injections, particularly those that have easily palpable landmarks. Others contend that accuracy is improved in even routine injections. There has yet to be a widespread consensus regarding which specific procedures are appropriate for ultrasound guidance. It is clear that it should be considered in circumstances where needle accuracy is needed for efficacy, safety, and/or visualization of the tissue effects of the procedure.

PLANNING THE PROCEDURE

Appropriate advanced planning will help ensure smooth execution of the procedure. A checklist of materials and equipment to be used should be reviewed in advance (Table 14.1). Sufficient time should be taken to inspect and establish that the correct medication and dosage is available. The needle

TABLE 14.1 Equipment and Materials for Ultrasound Guided Procedures

Medications (thoroughly examined for correct labeling and dosage)

Appropriate size and length needles

Local anesthetic (when needed)

Ultrasound machine with appropriate transducer (linear or curvilinear)

Skin preparation (sterilization) material

Gauge

Dressing or bandages

Sterilization material for the transducer or transducer cover

Gloves

Sterile drapes (when needed)

gauge and length should be appropriate for the procedure planned. There must be adequate length to reach the target. This includes a needle for a local anesthetic when needed.

Scanning the area of the procedure should be done in advance. This allows image optimization with the ultrasound machine as well as precisely determining the depth of the target for approach planning (Figure 14.1). A consideration for approach planning should be minimizing anisotropy of the needle. There is

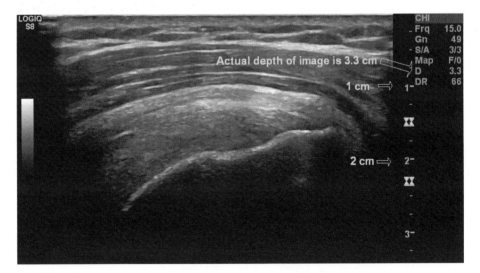

FIGURE 14.1 Sonogram demonstrating use of the measuring tool to determine the depth of the image. The sonogram is a long-axis view of the supraspinatus tendon. The depth of the entire image is shown. The markers to the right are also available to determine the depth at each level of the image in centimeters. Most ultrasound machines have measurement tools of this nature. They should be used in the prescan to determine the precise depth of the intended target in advance.

greater conspicuity when the incident ultrasound beam is more orthogonal to the needle (Figure 14.2). The needle is particularly more difficult to see when a steep angle is used for approaching deeper targets. For this reason, beginning the needle approach somewhat further from the target will facilitate a more perpendicular position and better needle visualization (Figure 14.3).

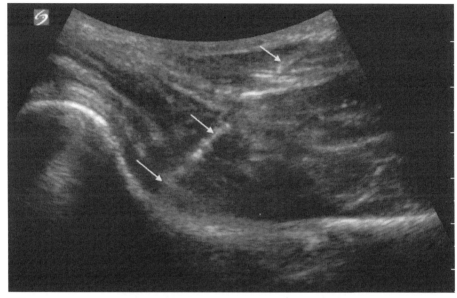

(A)

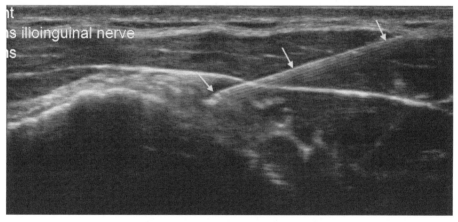

(B)

FIGURE 14.2 Sonograms demonstrating the effect of needle anisotropy with in-plane views of the needle. The image in (A) shows a long-axis view of the anterior hip. Note the more difficult needle visualization (yellow arrows) of a deeper injection. The image in (B) shows the improved conspicuity of a more superficial needle (yellow arrows). A needle that is more perpendicular to the incident sound beam is more easily visualized. Anisotropic artifact of deeper injections can be improved by initiating the injection further from the target to create a more perpendicular trajectory. The examiner can also use heel-to-toe rock of the transducer, or beam direction or steering, if available on the equipment, to increase the angle of incidence of the sound waves in relation to the needle.

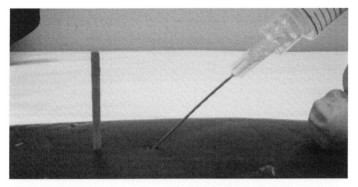

(A)

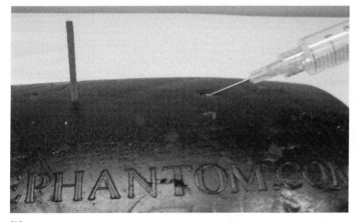

(B)

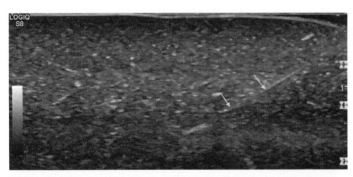

(C)

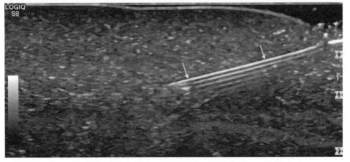

(D)

FIGURE 14.3 Pictures and sonograms demonstrating different needle approaches for the same target. The picture in (A) shows a steep trajectory toward the target. The picture in (B) shows an approach to the same target from a greater distance to apply a more orthogonal approach in relation to the transducer. The sonogram in (C) demonstrates the appearance of the needle (yellow arrow) from a steeper approach. The sonogram in (D) shows an in-plane view of the same needle (yellow arrows) with an approach that is more perpendicular to the needle. The disadvantage of this approach is that it results in the needle traversing through tissue over a greater length to reach the same target. The advantage is that it allows better visualization of the needle.

When approaching a very superficial target, an oblique standoff of piled up sterile gel on one end of the transducer can allow visualization of the needle prior to contact with the skin (Figure 14.4).

Scanning prior to the procedure provides help distinguishing undesirable areas for avoidance (Figure 14.5). During this time, the settings on the ultrasound machine should be reviewed including appropriate depth, focal zone placement, and frequency for optimization of the area to be visualized (see Chapter 4).

In addition to preparing the skin, antiseptic preparation of the transducer surface or a sterile transducer cover should be used to avoid contaminating the injection field. Use of alcohol-based chlorhexidine is preferred over povidone-iodine by some centers for skin preparation. Alcohol can

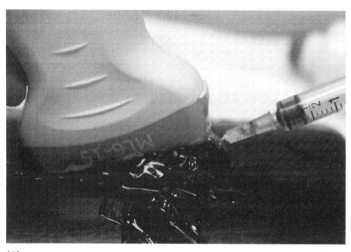

(A)

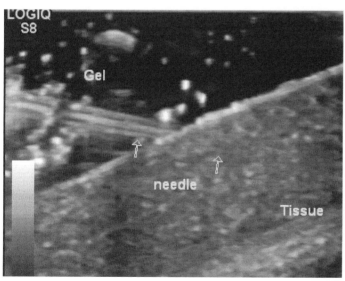

(B)

FIGURE 14.4 Demonstration of using a large amount of transducer gel to create an oblique standoff (A). This is reflected by the sonogram in (B). The oblique standoff of transducer gel allows visualization of the needle prior to making contact with the skin. This is particularly helpful when the target is a very superficial structure.

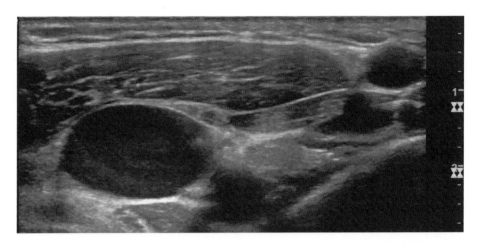

FIGURE 14.5 Sonogram demonstrating an example of an area where prescan planning and live guidance can help avoid undesirable placement of the needle. The image is an area of the neck with multiple neurovascular structures that could be avoided with proper technique.

potentially have adverse effect on the transducer crystals, so obtaining information from the manufacturer should be done prior to use of any substance with the transducer.

Use of sterile probe covers can alleviate the need to sterilize the transducer surface (Figure 14.6). This is a good option because it allows free movement of the transducer in the field to optimize tissue and needle conspicuity.

The "no touch" method can also be used. This is accomplished by keeping the nonsterile transducer completely out of the sterile field (Figure 14.7). Although potentially time saving, this method presents the problem of the limitation of transducer movement in situations when the needle is difficult

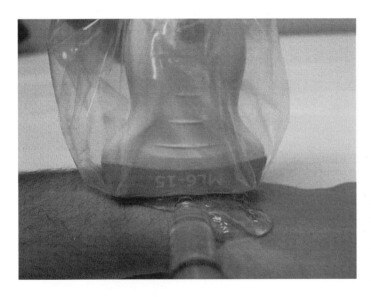

FIGURE 14.6 Picture of a transducer with a sterile cover. The cover allows movement of the transducer in the area of the procedure without contaminating the sterile field.

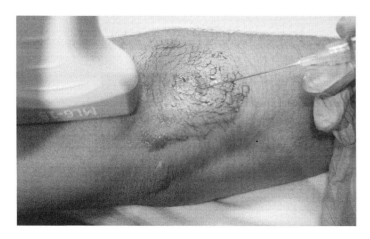

FIGURE 14.7 Picture demonstrating the "no touch" method of performing a sterile injection. The image is created at an angle to the target and the transducer is kept out of the sterile field.

to visualize. It also provides a greater risk of sterile field contamination, particularly in less experienced practitioners.

The procedure should also be explained to the patient during the preparation period providing "informed consent." It is also reasonable to explain the benefit and potentially improved accuracy of ultrasound guidance to the patient. Some patients may have had similar injections without guidance and be surprised by the additional preparation time. Anxiety can be alleviated with an explanation that the additional preparation provides a more accurate injection.

Consideration should also be given to the orientation of the transducer and needle relative to the anatomic target. The terms *short axis* and *long axis* refer to the position of the transducer relative to the anatomic target (Figure 14.8). The terms *in-plane* and *out-of-plane* refer to the orientation of the needle relative to the transducer. With in-plane orientation, the needle is parallel to the transducer. With out-of-plane orientation, the needle is perpendicular to the transducer (Figure 14.9). In-plane orientation is generally preferred for most injections for the advantage of visualization of the entire needle approach and needle tip (Figure 14.10). Out-of-plane injections can be used effectively in some circumstances, particularly when the target is superficial and close to the point of skin insertion. The needle in an out-of-plane view will appear as a hyperechoic dot (Figure 14.11). This view has the disadvantage of only showing a small cross section of the needle and not facilitating reliable visualization of the needle tip.

The arrangement of the patient and injection field in relationship to the ultrasound machine should also be considered in advance. Having the ultrasound screen in direct line with the needle and transducer will facilitate an easier injection by allowing visualization of all of these components without having to avert gaze away from the needle (Figure 5.8). Consideration of which hand will hold the transducer and which will be used to perform the injection should also be determined in advance. Many practitioners prefer to stabilize the transducer with the nondominant hand and perform

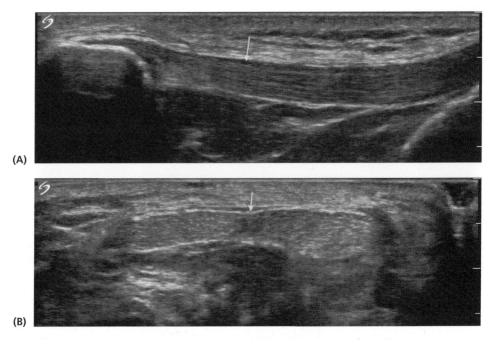

(A)

(B)

FIGURE 14.8 Sonograms demonstrating the appearance of the patellar tendon (yellow arrow) in long axis (A) and short axis (B).

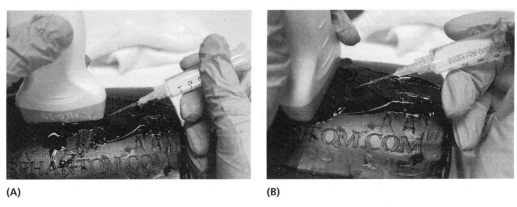

(A)   (B)

FIGURE 14.9 Pictures demonstrating the orientation of an in-plane (A) and out-of-plane (B) position of the needle relative to the transducer.

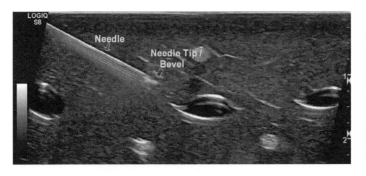

FIGURE 14.10 Sonogram demonstrating an in-plane view of a needle. This orientation is generally preferable for most injections as it allows visualization of the needle tip throughout its trajectory.

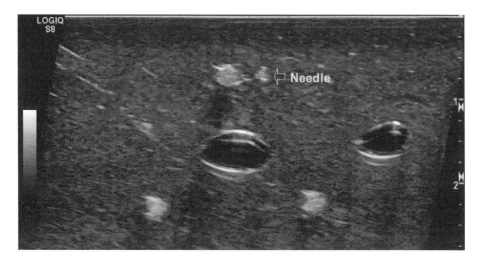

FIGURE 14.11 Sonogram demonstrating an out-of-plane view of the needle. This orientation is sometimes more challenging because the needle tip and length of the needle are not seen. In this view, the needle will appear as a hyperechoic dot when it moves into the field. It can be used successfully for needle introduction into small spaces over short distances.

the injection with the dominant hand. The time spent doing a plan of the injection approach with the preprocedure scan can provide considerable rewards for improving the ease of the injection.

PERFORMING THE INJECTION

Once the appropriate planning has been completed, the needle should be inserted with the same trajectory as determined during the prescanning period. Once the target has been identified on ultrasound, the needle must be directed toward the center of the transducer. One should resist staring at the screen to find the needle while not referring back to the needle position relative to the transducer. The ultrasound beam is thin and any deviation from the center of the transducer will result in an inability to visualize the needle with in-plane injections.

Anisotropy can make the needle difficult to visualize even when it has been effectively placed under the transducer with in-plane approach. For this reason, the more perpendicular the needle is to the transducer position, the greater the conspicuity. This should also be considered when planning the injection. Using heel-to-toe rocking and toggling can sometimes increase needle visibility (Figure 14.12). Many ultrasound machines have settings that allow alteration of the beam from the transducer to create a more orthogonal approach of the incident beam relative to the needle position (Figure 14.13).

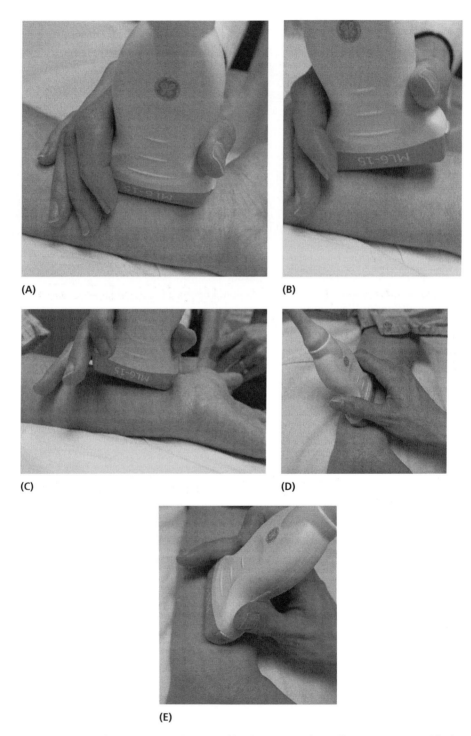

FIGURE 14.12 Pictures demonstrating the use of heel-to-toe and toggling maneuvers with the transducer to eliminate anisotropic artifact. Image (A) shows the transducer in a relatively neutral position with respect to the underlying tissue. Images (B) and (C) show the changes in position in a heel-to-toe rock. The images in (D) and (E) show the changes in position in toggling. These maneuvers are designed to change the direction of the incident beam to create an incident angle to as close to 90° as possible to the object being observed.

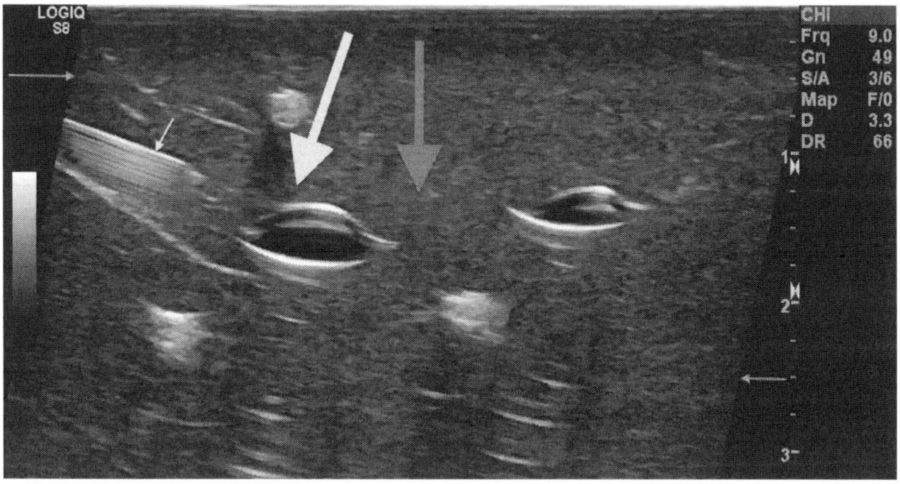

FIGURE 14.13 Sonogram of an in-plane view of a needle (small yellow arrow) using directional change or "beam steering" to change the angle of incidence of the sound waves. This technique allows the examiner to maintain even contact on the skin with the transducer but alters the beam in a favorable direction to increase the angle of incidence to the needle. The large blue arrow indicates the direction of the incident sound waves without this feature. The large yellow arrow shows the direction of the incident sound waves with this feature activated. The change in direction of the margins (orange arrows) indicates the beam steering is activated. Altering the beam to create a more perpendicular approach in relation to the needle position allows for better needle visualization.

The needle should not be advanced if the tip is not visualized. Other maneuvers that can help to visualize the needle tip include jiggling the needle tip back and forth and rotating the needle bevel. When jiggling, the needle is rapidly moved back and forth in relatively small amounts. This movement often increases conspicuity of the tip. Rotating the needle will often help identify the tip because of the asymmetric shape of the bevel.

With out-of-plane orientation the needle is generally easier to visualize, however, only a cross-sectional view is seen. Caution must be used with this approach because the needle appearance is roughly the same regardless of the position of the needle tip (Figure 14.14). The tip is confirmed by the first appearance of the hyperechoic dot as the needle is advanced into the tissue field. In situations where the tip appears at the incorrect depth, the needle should be partially withdrawn and readvanced to the appropriate depth.

Needle reverberation artifact can distort the image of the needle (Figure 14.15). This occurs as a result of the incident sound beam bouncing back and forth between the transducer and the high impedance needle (Figure 13.7). Understanding of this artifact can prevent confusion with this distorted image.

Documentation of the ultrasound-guided procedure should, at a minimum, include an image of the tissue target. An image showing the needle in the proper position is preferable. There should also be documentation of the

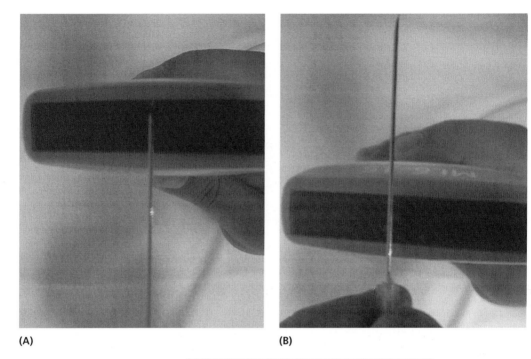

(A)   (B)

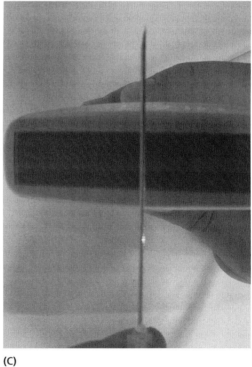

(C)

FIGURE 14.14 Pictures demonstrating the potential out-of-plane position of a needle relative to the transducer that all display the same ultrasound image (A)–(C). All three positions will appear as a single hyperechoic dot. For this reason, caution must be used to maintain the location of the needle tip when using the out-of-plane orientation.

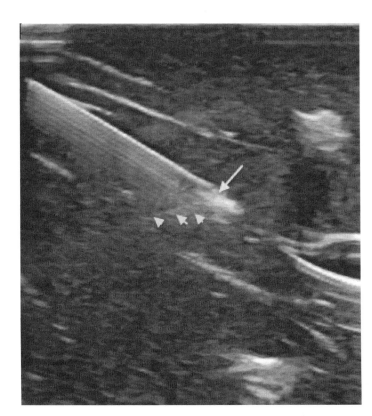

FIGURE 14.15 Sonogram demonstrating needle reverberation artifact. The needle is shown in in-plane view. The needle tip is identified by the yellow arrow and the reverberation artifact is identified by the blue arrowheads. It is important to recognize what portion of the image represents artifact for reliable needle placement.

need for the procedure including an explanation of the need for ultrasound guidance. Becoming proficient at ultrasound guidance requires practice. Using objects such as turkey breasts with placed targets or practice tools such as Blue Phantoms (Figure 14.16) can enhance skills before performing injections in live clinical situations.

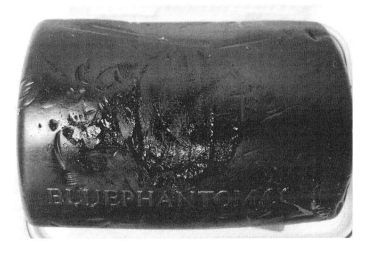

FIGURE 14.16 Picture of an example of a commercial practice tool that can be used to practice guided injections.

REMEMBER ···

1) Preprocedure scanning should always be performed to assess for any undesirable areas and plan the depth and precise location of the target.
2) The transducer should be positioned so that the direction of the incident sound waves is perpendicular to the needle as much as possible to minimize anisotropic artifact.
3) In-plane needle orientation is generally preferable to visualize the advancement of the needle tip. When out-of-plane orientation is used, great care is needed to establish when the tip of the needle first arrives in the field.

BIBLIOGRAPHY

1. Daley E, Bajaj S, Bisson L, Cole B. Improving injections accuracy of the elbow, knee, and shoulder: does injection site and imaging make a difference? A systemic review. *Am J Sports Med*. 2011;39:656–662.

2. Lento PA, Strakowski JA. The use of ultrasound in guiding musculoskeletal interventional procedures. *Phys Med Rehabil Clin N Am*. 2010;21:559–583.

3. Malanga G, Mautner K. *Atlas of Ultrasound-Guided Musculoskeletal Injections*. New York, NY: McGraw-Hill; 2013.

4. Peck E, Lai JK, Pawlina W, Smith J. Accuracy of ultrasound guided versus palpation-guided acromioclavicular joint injections: a cadaveric study. *PM&R*. 2010;2(9):817–821.

5. Smith J, Finnoff JT. Diagnostic and interventional musculoskeletal ultrasound: part 1. Fundamentals. *PM&R*. 2009;1(1):64–75.

CHAPTER 15

Developing a Clinical Practice

As knowledge in musculoskeletal ultrasound training progresses, the next step is to utilize it in clinical practice. This is done by obtaining adequate equipment, developing scanning and interpreting skills, and taking the necessary steps to integrate these techniques into improvement in patient care.

OBTAINING AN ULTRASOUND MACHINE

Obtaining an ultrasound machine is the first and necessary step toward developing a clinical practice. It is virtually impossible to adequately progress without the machine for practice as well as clinical use. It is also typically the largest step a practitioner will make, as it requires a considerable financial investment. Currently, machines can vary in cost between twenty and two hundred thousand dollars. The quality of the machine tends to parallel the cost. Despite this, the machines have continued to improve to the extent that the lower cost portable machines can provide a high quality image that can easily be used in clinical practice.

There are a number of quality companies that make ultrasound machines that can be used for musculoskeletal medicine. It is prudent for a potential buyer to "test drive" different types of machines to determine the best choice for an individual practice. This can be done at meetings, by contacting the vendors directly for demonstrations, or finding other practitioners with a machine to assess. The desirable features of an ultrasound machine are dependent on the particular needs of the individual. For virtually all practitioners, however, the machine should have a high-resolution broadband linear transducer, be able to provide a high quality image and have digital storage. Determining the best company to use for ultrasound purchase is also individualized but it is advised to investigate which companies have the best customer service.

DEVELOP SCANNING AND INTERPRETING SKILLS

Practitioners have traditionally had to seek out opportunities to develop skills in musculoskeletal ultrasound. Until recently, formal training in this discipline was not available in most residency programs. As the field has grown, an increasing number of learning opportunities have developed that include didactic courses, instructional books, journal articles, and online videos. There are also a growing number of instructors that can teach their experience. Seeking out other individuals with the same interest can also be invaluable. Regular communication with a network of other practitioners doing similar evaluations can provide practical insight that might not be found in a typical journal or textbook. There is no substitute to practice time with the ultrasound machine.

Attend Hands-On Courses

There are a number of courses available that are put on by multiple organizations that teach both musculoskeletal and neuromuscular ultrasound. These can be found as both stand-alone courses and components of larger meetings for various medical disciplines. This includes sports medicine, physical medicine and rehabilitation, radiology, rheumatology, neurology, and a host of other musculoskeletal practitioners. These courses allow instruction and direct teaching from experts in the field and in many cases, hands-on instruction with supervision and feedback. The number of courses has grown to the extent that there is an available opportunity virtually every month of the year. Many are tailored for different experience levels so the degree of difficulty should be determined prior to enrolling.

An additional advantage of attending ultrasound meetings and courses is the opportunity to meet and network with other individuals with similar academic and practice interests. Much can be learned simply from hearing the experiences from other traveling the same road. Courses are an excellent way to learn or refine new skills.

Learn the Anatomy

There is no substitute for detailed knowledge of anatomy when performing ultrasound evaluations. It takes considerable practice to reliably construct an understanding of three-dimensional anatomy using two-dimensional gray-scale images. Continually practicing scanning on friends, family, and anyone that will tolerate it will help develop this skill. Returning to an anatomy lab can provide great rewards for further understanding. Having anatomy books available and using them frequently is a mandatory exercise for improvement.

INCORPORATION OF ULTRASOUND INTO A CLINICAL PRACTICE

Supervision in Practice

Although expert supervision in hands-on course can be valuable, there is no replacement for expert review in a true clinical setting. While this is typical for residents in training, it is often more difficult for a learner who is out in clinical practice. Finding experienced mentors with experience in ultrasound can be very helpful.

Limit the Scope of the Examinations Until Sufficient Experience Is Obtained

The field of musculoskeletal ultrasound is very broad. For most, it requires years of training and practice to acquire proficiency in multiple body regions. It is preferable to limit the scope of the clinical practice initially to areas of proficiency rather than provide erroneous diagnostic information by commenting on anatomy that has not been adequately mastered. The clinical practice can be progressively expanded as skills continue to improve. It is also helpful to obtain a clinical checklist of important structures to evaluate for each body region when first beginning in practice.

Seek Accreditation When Available

Accreditation and certification are available through some organizations, both as an individual and as a laboratory where the testing is performed. Although gaining accreditation and/or certification through various societies might not be recognized by all third party payers, having some recognition for training competency can be helpful in many circumstances.

Use Ultrasound as an Extension of the Clinical History and Examination

Musculoskeletal ultrasound images should never be used in isolation by clinical practitioners. The findings should always be correlated with a reasonably detailed history and physical examination. Pathology can often be found in musculoskeletal structures that have little relation to the patient's complaint. Having a good understanding of the proper clinical context of the findings will dramatically improve utility of the ultrasound examination.

The use of ultrasound should enhance clinical musculoskeletal assessment, not make it more challenging. One of the sure-fire methods of improving skills in musculoskeletal ultrasound is to improve overall knowledge in musculoskeletal medicine. Similarly, the use of ultrasound for guided injections should improve interventional skills that have already been developed.

Know Your Limitations

There will always be limitations to any diagnostic modality and always limitations of anyone's individual skills. The practitioner should be aware of these limitations and seek help with other diagnostic modalities or obtain consultations when appropriate. No single diagnostic test can solve every medical problem.

Stay Current

The field of musculoskeletal ultrasound has been changing rapidly with progressive advances in techniques and imaging capabilities. It requires continued effort to remain current with the evolving knowledge base but there is a multitude of available resources. This includes textbooks, websites, podcasts, journal articles, and didactic lectures. Becoming involved with organizations devoted to the advancement of musculoskeletal ultrasound is invaluable.

CONCLUSION

Beginning the process of developing a musculoskeletal practice can appear intimidating at first, but using a disciplined approach of mastering the material will add confidence. Taking advantage of available educational resources, networking with other interested practitioners, finding experienced mentors, and most importantly regular practice will lead to continued improvement. Musculoskeletal ultrasound can be a very rewarding discipline and often provides great patient satisfaction and leads to improved patient care (Figure 15.1).

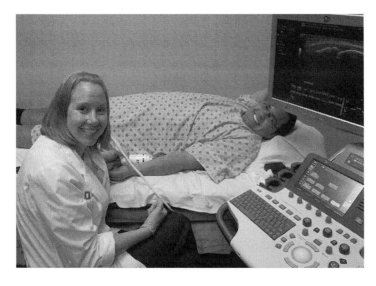

FIGURE 15.1 Picture demonstrating a happy and successful musculoskeletal ultrasound practice.

Index

absorption attenuation process, 12
Achilles tendon, 71, 73, 116, 122
acoustic impedance, 7, 14
  of bone, 115
acromial–clavicular joint, 117
acute latissimus dorsi muscle strain
    injury, 90
acute strains, 89
adequate tissue penetration, 45
adipose tissue, 120
advanced controls, 39
AIIS. *See* anterior inferior iliac spine
alcohol, 39
alcohol-based chlorhexidine, use of, 169
A-mode, ultrasound imaging modes, 20
anechoic lumen of superficial vein,
    137–138
angle of incidence, 7, 9–11
anisotropy, artifacts, 9, 126, 155–156, 173
  on biceps brachii tendon, 47
  of deeper injections, 167
  minimize, 47–48
anterior inferior iliac spine (AIIS), 74, 78
anticoagulation therapy, 137–138
architecture, muscle, 81–85
arteries, 129–131
artifacts, 155, 163
  anisotropy, 155–156
  inadequate conduction medium,
    156–157
  posterior acoustic enhancement, 159–160

posterior acoustic shadowing, 158–159
  reverberation artifact, 161–162
attenuation, 163
  sound waves of, 4, 7
    absorption process, 12
    reflection process, 7–10
    refraction process, 10–12
attenuation coefficient, 7

backscatter, 12
Baker's cyst, linear measurement of, 35
bandwidth of transducers, 4
biceps brachii muscle, long-axis and
    short-axis views of, 86
biceps brachii tendon, 42, 69, 70
  anisotropy on, 47
bipennate muscle, 81, 83
Blue Phantoms, 177
B-mode ultrasound, 61
  imaging modes, 20, 21
bone, 115–119
  erosions and hypertrophy, 119
bone shadow, 115
bony landmarks, 116
border, masses
  characteristics of, 143
  nature of, 143–144
brachial artery, 129, 131
brachial plexus, 36
broad bandwidth transducers, 4

bursae, 127–128
bursal enlargement, 127
bursitis, 127

cartilage, 123–125
caution, 175
cellulitis, 121, 123
chronic muscle strains, 89
claustrophobia, 1
clinical practice, developing
  incorporation of ultrasound, 181–182
  scanning and interpreting skills, 180–181
  ultrasound machine, obtaining, 179–180
color Doppler, 32, 33, 62–63, 129–132,
    134–135, 147
  flash artifact with, 65
  versus power Doppler, 63–67
comet tail artifact, 162
complex olecranon bursitis, 128
conduction gel, 54, 156, 157
conspicuity
  degree of, 116
  of needle, 155–156
conventional gray scale, 131
conventional venous Doppler
    evaluation, 132
convergent muscles, 82, 83
convergent pattern of deltoid, 84
coracoacromial ligament, 126
curvilinear transducer, 18–20
cyst, 146

deep venous thrombosis, 132
degree of conspicuity, 116
deltoid, convergent pattern of, 84
denervation, 94–95
depth
  selecting appropriate, 43–44
  setting, 21–22
diffuse reflection, specular reflection
    versus, 8
direct piezoelectric effect, 3
direct tracing method, 106, 107
documentation of ultrasound-guided
    procedure, 175
Doppler imaging, 1, 32–33, 129, 130, 132,
    147–148
  color Doppler, 62–63
  power Doppler, 61–62

for tibial artery and veins identification,
    99, 102
Doppler ultrasound tendons, 76, 79
DVD burner, 37
dynamic abnormalities, 1
dynamic capabilities of ultrasound, 87
dynamic visualization, 1

echo, 3
echotexture, 144–146
edema, 121
emitted sound wave, frequency of, 4
ergonomics, 56–58
excessive pressure, with transducer, 52, 53
excessive refraction and attenuation, 163
external trauma, 92

fasciculus, 81
fat, 120–123
fat necrosis, 121
fibrillar pattern of tendons, 71, 72
fibrocartilage, 123, 125
flash artifact with color Doppler, 65
focal neuropathies, 109
focal zone, selecting appropriate, 46
footprint transducers, 20
foreign bodies
  glass, 153
  introduction, 149–151
  metal, 152
  wood, 152
frequency
  control, 23
  selecting appropriate, 45
  of sound waves, 4–6
fusiform, 82, 83

gain, selecting appropriate, 46
ganglion cyst, 146
gel and standoff pads, 38
glass, foreign body, 153
gray scale gain, 23–24
gray scale image, 61
gray scale mapping, selecting, 47
grip, transducer, 51, 52

harmonic frequency waves, 13
heel-to-toe maneuver, 54

heel-to-toe rocking
  needle, 173, 174
  of transducer, 55
hematomas, 89, 90
hernias, 92–93
Hertz (Hz), 4
heterogeneous postsurgical scar, 120
higher frequency linear transducers, 18
high-flow vascular structure, 66
high-frequency broadband
    transducers, 18
high-frequency musculoskeletal
    ultrasound, 17
high-frequency ultrasound, 2
high-frequency waveforms, 5
high-resolution broadband high-frequency
    transducers, development of, 2
high-resolution broadband linear
    transducer, 179
hyaline cartilage, 123, 125
hyper, 144
hyperechoic (bright) connective tissue, 81
hyperechoic fibrillar appearance, 126
hyperechoic muscle layer, 121
hyperechoic septa, 120
hyperechoic (bright) signal, 14, 48
hyperechoic thrombosis, 137
hypo, 144
hypoechoic appearance of tendon
    fibers, 156
hypoechoic hyaline cartilage, 124
hypoechoic lobules, 120
hypoechoic muscle fibers, 82
hypoechoic (dark) nerve fascicles, normal
    nerve, 99, 100
hypoechoic ring of reactive tissue, 149
Hz. *See* Hertz

image optimization
  depth, selecting appropriate, 43–44
  focal zone, selecting appropriate, 46
  frequency, selecting appropriate, 45
  gain, selecting appropriate, 46
  gray scale mapping, selecting, 47
  image with transducer, centering, 42–43
  labels, appropriate, 48
  minimize anisotropic artifact, 47–48
  oriented image, 41–42
image storage, 36–37
image with transducer, centering, 42–43

imaging masses
  border, nature of, 143–144
  compressibility of, 146
  echotexture of, 144–146
  relationship to surrounding tissue,
    146–147
  size of, 141–143
  systematic approach to, 141
  vascularity of, 147–148
imaging modalities, 115
imaging muscle, 81
  architecture, 81–85
  pathology
    anomolous, congenitally absent, and
      accessory muscles, 96–97
    denervation, 94–95
    hernias, 92–93
    myopathy, 95–96
    postsurgical or traumatic alteration, 92
    strains, 88–91
  techniques, 85–87
inadequate conduction medium, 156–157
incident sound waves, 9, 10, 47
  propagation of, 12
inflammatory arthropathies, 119
informed consent, 171
infraspinatus muscle, short-axis view of, 95
injection, performing, 173–177
inner epineurium, 99
in-plane view of needle, 171, 172, 175
instrument, cleaning, 39
intercalated fibrillar pattern, normal nerve,
    99, 100
inverse piezoelectric effect, 3

jiggling, 175
jugular vein, short-axis view of, 159
juxtapose sequential images, 33

Kager's fat pad, 122
knowledge of artifacts, 155

labeling, 36
labels, appropriate, 48
ligaments, 126–127
linear broadband transducer, 4, 18
linear transducers, 17–19
Lister's tubercle, 116, 137–138
long axis of transducer, 171

long-axis view of supraspinatus
    tendon, 166
low-frequency waveforms, 5
low-grade muscle strain, 89

mapping, 28–32
marking tool, 34–35
masses, imaging
  border, nature of, 143–144
  compressibility of, 146
  echotexture of, 144–146
  relationship to surrounding tissue,
      146–147
  size of, 141–143
  systematic approach to, 141
  vascularity of, 147–148
measurement tool, 34–35
medial gastrocnemius, 137–138
median nerve, 11
medical diagnostic ultrasound, 20
medical disciplines, 180
megahertz (MHz), 4
metal, foreign body, 152
MHz. *See* megahertz
minimize anisotropic artifact, 47–48
M-mode, ultrasound imaging
      modes, 20, 21
mucosal bursae, 128
multipennate muscle, 81, 83
muscle echotexture, 95
muscle fibers
  bundle of, 83
  diameter, 81
  echotexture, 89
  irregular disruption of, 92
muscle herniation, long-axis view of, 93
muscle, imaging, 81
  architecture, 81–85
  pathology
    anomolous, congenitally absent, and
        accessory muscles, 96–97
    denervation, 94–95
    hernias, 92–93
    myopathy, 95–96
    postsurgical or traumatic
        alteration, 92
    strains, 88–91
  techniques, 85–87
muscle movement, 87
musculoskeletal assessment, 120

musculoskeletal ultrasound, 1, 2, 182
  artifacts in, 155
  evaluations, 18
  examination, 2
  images, 181
  reverberation artifact, 161–162
  scanning, 32
  sure-fire methods of improving skills
      in, 182
myopathy, 95–96

needle
  anisotropy, effect of, 167
  approaches, 168
  conspicuity of, 155–156
  in-plane view of, 172, 175
  out-of-plane view of, 173
  reverberation artifact, 175, 177
neovascularization, 66
nerves
  architecture of, 99–103
  artery and veins, 101
  entrapment, illustration of, 109
  hypoechoic (dark) nerve fascicles, 99, 100
  intercalated fibrillar pattern, 99, 100
  pathology, 109–113
  uninterrupted fascicular pattern, 99, 100
nerve scanning techniques, 103–108
  anatomic landmarks, 103, 105
  anisotropy use, 104
  cross-sectional area measurements,
      106, 107
  diameter measurement, 108
  direct tracing method, 106, 107
  transducer pressure, 105
neurogenic atrophy, 94, 95
nondisplaced fibular fracture, 119
nonvascular settings, 66
normal Achilles tendon, 156
normal fibrillar architecture of tendon, 156
normal hyaline cartilage, 123
normal scapholunate ligament, 127
normal skin, disorders of, 120
"no touch" method, 170, 171
novice scanners, 51

oblique standoff of transducer gel, 169
olecranon spur, 118
optimal reflection, 9

orthogonal planes, 141
outer epineurium, 99
out-of-plane injections, 171
out-of-plane view of needle, 173

parallel muscles, 81–83
patellar tendon (PT), 70, 72, 73, 122, 172
pennate muscles, 81
peripheral nerves
    appearance of, 109
    components of, 101
    focal median neuropathy, 110, 112
    nerve entrapment, illustration of, 109
    nerve swelling, 109, 110
    pathology determination, 110, 111
    ultrasound, 99, 112–113
piezoelectric effect, 3
plain film radiography, 149
posterior acoustic enhancement, 159–160
posterior acoustic shadowing, 158–159
posterior artifact, 149
postsurgical/traumatic alteration, 92
potential out-of-plane position of
        needle, 176
power Doppler, 32–33, 61–62, 76, 129, 130,
        132, 147
    color Doppler versus, 63–67
PT. See patellar tendon
pulse, 3

quadrilateral-shaped pronator
        quadratus, 85
quadrilateral-type muscles, 82, 83

radial artery pseudoaneurysm, 131
real-time imaging, 1
real-time visualization of needle
        motion, 1
reflection attenuation process, 7–10
refraction attenuation process, 10–12
reverberation artifact, 161–162
reverse piezoelectric effect, 3, 17
ring-down artifact, 162

scanning techniques, 51–56
    for tendons, 71–75
scapholunate ligament (SLL), 126
scatter, 12–13

SCM. See sternocleidomastoid
short-axis view
    of jugular vein, 159
    of muscle, 81
    of transducer, 171
side-to-side comparison imaging, 48
single transducer, 20
skeletal muscle, 81
    components of, 83
skin, 119–120
SLL. See scapholunate ligament
Snell's law, 10
sound beam, 11
sound waves, 3, 66
    attenuation. See attenuation, sound
        waves of
    frequency of, 4–6
    harmonic frequency, 13
    propagation, 10
    scatter, 12–13
    speed of, 13–14
    transmission, speed of, 13–14
speckle, 12
specular reflection, 7
    versus diffuse reflection, 8
split screen image, 33–34
standoff pads, gel and, 38
"starry night" appearance of
        muscle, 81, 82
sterile probe covers, use of, 170
sterile transducer, 169
sternocleidomastoid (SCM), 94
strains, 88–91
stress maneuvers, 126
subacromial–subdeltoid
        bursa, 127, 128
substantial knowledge base,
        development of, 2
superficial musculoskeletal
        applications, 4
superficial vein, anechoic lumen of,
        137–138
superficial venous thrombosis, 137
supraspinatus tendon, long-axis
        view of, 166
sure-fire methods, 182
synovial bursae, 128
synovial-lined sac, 127
synovitis, 61
    effect of, 67

tendons, 155
  anisotropic artifact, 74
  calcification, 76, 77
  Doppler ultrasound, 76, 79
  fibrillar architecture of, 69, 70
  fibrillar pattern of, 71, 72
  heel-to-toe rocking maneuvers, 74, 75
  pathology of, 76–79
  rectus femoris from AIIS, 74, 78
  scanning technique for, 71–75
  side-to-side comparisons, 76, 79
  structure of, 69–70
  toggling, 74, 75
TGC. *See* time gain compensation
three-dimensional anatomy, 180
time gain compensation (TGC), 24–28
tissue properties
  acoustic impedance, 14
  speed of sound wave, 13–14
toggling, 156, 173, 174
  tendons, 74, 75
  of transducer, 54
traditional transducer, 17
transducer, 4, 17–20, 41, 47, 62, 85, 86,
    126, 170
  centering image with, 42–43
  excessive pressure with, 52, 53
  long axis of, 171
  pressure, 105, 129, 132–134
  short axis of, 171
  skill, 42
  traditional, 17
  ultrasound, 39
  use of, 51–56
transducer gel, oblique standoff of, 169
trauma, 121
traumatic alteration, 92
2D-mode, ultrasound imaging
    modes, 20–21

ulnar nerve, 103
ultrasonography, inadequate conduction
    medium, 156

ultrasound, 81, 116, 141
  advantages of, 1
  into clinical practice, incorporation of,
    181–182
  dynamic capabilities of, 87
  evaluation, positioning for
    performing, 57
  foreign bodies, 149, 153
  high-frequency, 2
  identification of muscle
    strains, 88
  imaging, 4, 123
  imaging modes, 20–21
  incorporation of, 2
  machine, obtaining, 179–180
  peripheral nerves on, 99, 109, 112–113
  physics used in, 3
  piezoelectric effect, 3
  pulses, 21
  sound waves. *See* sound waves
  tendons, 69, 76
  tissue properties, 13–14
  transducer, 39
  waves, 115
ultrasound beam, 173
  focal zone of, 46
ultrasound-guided injection, 165
  indications for, 165
  performing, 58, 173–177
  procedure planning, 165–173
ultrasound-guided procedures
  documentation of, 175
  equipment and materials for, 166
uninterrupted fascicular pattern, normal
    nerve, 99, 100

vascular structure, 146
veins, 132–138
venous thrombosis, 132, 137–138
volar forearm, short-axis view of, 87

wood, foreign body, 152

Printed in the United States
By Bookmasters